The Renal System

Commissioning Editor: Timothy Horne
Development Editor: Lulu Stader
Project Manager: Janaki Srinivasan Kumar
Designer/Design Direction: Charles Gray
Illustration Manager: Gillian Richards

SYSTEMS OF THE BODY

The Renal System

BASIC SCIENCE AND CLINICAL CONDITIONS

SECOND EDITION

Michael J. Field

MD, BS, BSc(Hons), FRACP
Professor of Medicine and Associate Dean
Royal North Shore Hospital
St Leonards, NSW, Australia

University of Nottingham
at Derby Library

Carol A. Pollock

MB, BS, PhD, FRACP
Professor of Medicine and Area Chair of Research
Royal North Shore Hospital
St Leonards, NSW, Australia

David C. Harris

MD, BS, FRACP
Professor of Medicine and Associate Dean
Westmead Hospital
Westmead, NSW, Australia

All of Discipline of Medicine, University of Sydney, Australia

Illustrations by Robert Britton

CHURCHILL
LIVINGSTONE

ELSEVIER

EDINBURGH LONDON NEW YORK OXFORD PHILADELPHIA ST LOUIS SYDNEY TORONTO 2010

CHURCHILL
LIVINGSTONE
ELSEVIER

First Edition Harcourt Publishers Limited 2001.
Second Edition © 2010, Elsevier Limited. All rights reserved.

ISBN: 978-0-7020-3371-1

British Library Cataloguing in Publication Data
A catalogue record for this book is available from the British Library

Library of Congress Cataloging in Publication Data
A catalog record for this book is available from the Library of Congress

1006101662

Notice
Knowledge and best practice in this field are constantly changing. As new research and experience broaden our knowledge, changes in practice, treatment and drug therapy may become necessary or appropriate. Readers are advised to check the most current information provided (i) on procedures featured or (ii) by the manufacturer of each product to be administered, to verify the recommended dose or formula, the method and duration of administration, and contraindications. It is the responsibility of the practitioner, relying on their own experience and knowledge of the patient, to make diagnoses, to determine dosages and the best treatment for each individual patient, and to take all appropriate safety precautions. To the fullest extent of the law, neither the Publisher nor the Authors assume any liability for any injury and/or damage to persons or property arising out of or related to any use of the material contained in this book.

The Publisher

Printed in China

Medical students, and indeed many practising doctors, have generally regarded learning about the normal kidney and its diseases as one of the more difficult areas in medicine. Many of the underlying concepts of normal structure and function may seem rather abstract, and the classification and manifestations of disease states can be confusing.

One of the reasons for this perceived difficulty in studying the kidney may be that the component disciplines have traditionally been presented largely in isolation from each other, so that the relationships between normal and abnormal structure and function, and the relevance of basic scientific descriptions to clinical problems, has not been made clear.

This book, like others in the Systems of the Body series, aims to guide beginning medical students in learning about the kidney by adopting a closely integrated approach. Each chapter is based around a clinical case scenario, and the process of working through the patient's problems leads to exploration of a variety of relevant material, drawn from the basic and clinical sciences as required. For example, in the first chapter, the presentation of a child with a probable urinary infection leads to consideration of the normal anatomy of the urinary tract and of developmental abnormalities which may predispose to urinary infection. At the same time, aspects of microbiology, antibiotic pharmacology, and modalities for imaging the urinary tract are dealt with, in context.

By this means, most of the important basic sciences relevant to understanding the structure, function and diseases of the renal system are covered, at a level appropriate to medical students in the first part of their course. The approach taken complements the philosophy of problem-based learning (PBL), which is being adopted by ever increasing numbers of medical schools throughout the world, though it should be equally useful to students enrolled in more conventional programs. Indeed, the book should in no way be seen as short-circuiting the process of self-directed learning which is at the heart of PBL-based courses, and it is expected that students will also consult conventional discipline-based textbooks and the medical literature to expand the horizons of their understanding of the subject-matter of the book.

In order to acknowledge that many students using this text will have had little clinical experience at this early stage of their course, we have provided a Glossary to define unfamiliar clinical terms used in the book (other than words which are explained within the context of the relevant chapter). Such terms are shown in bold in the text on their first occurrence.

While there are many developments in basic renal science, and many clinical conditions involving the kidney, which are not covered in this introductory book, we feel confident that students who master the material we have included here will be in a good position to take the study of the kidney further in their later undergraduate and postgraduate training.

. . .

In the years since this text first appeared, there have been many developments in basic science relevant to renal function, and some important advances in therapeutics and clinical care. However, the core knowledge structures which underpin the study of this system at medical student level have not undergone fundamental change; hence the design and essential content of the book has not been greatly altered for this second edition.

The authors have taken care to update information in some areas, to correct minor errors in the first edition, and to add some new illustrations. The opportunity has also been taken to incorporate some widely adopted changes in terminology, especially for acute renal failure, now referred to as acute kidney injury (AKI), and chronic renal failure, now chronic kidney disease (CKD). Some 'Interesting facts' relating to the material in the main text have been added in a number of places, in keeping with this feature of other volumes in the Systems of the Body series. Finally, three new chapters have been added, covering end-stage kidney disease and the replacement of renal function, pregnancy and the kidney, and renal masses and urinary tract tumours.

It is hoped that the new edition will continue to be found useful by medical students around the world.

ACKNOWLEDGEMENTS

It is a pleasure to acknowledge the enthusiasm and assistance of the publishers in producing this volume in the Systems of the Body series. In particular, the vision and leadership of Michael Parkinson, Commissioning Editor, and Timothy Horne, Publisher, and the attention to detail of Sarah Keer-Keer, Lynn Watt and Lulu Stader, Project Development Managers, were greatly appreciated.

A number of our colleagues assisted by offering suggestions for the improvement of the text, or by providing material for the illustrations. Dr George Kotsiou, of the Royal North Shore Hospital, Sydney, contributed to the microbiology sections of Chapter 1, while various photographic images were provided by colleagues at Concord Hospital, Westmead Hospital, Royal North Shore Hospital and the Department of Pathology, University of Sydney. For the second edition, specific thanks are due to Drs Kris Rasiah and Justin Vass (Department of Urology) and Dr Anthony Gill (Department of Anatomical Pathology, all of Royal North Shore Hospital) for assistance with the material for Chapter 13. We also thank Professor Robert Unwin for his helpful suggestions for the revised manuscript.

A special word of thanks is due to Beverley Smith, who assisted with preparation of the manuscript, and, as is traditional (but also appropriate), we would all like to acknowledge the patience shown by our families during the period in which this book was being written.

CONTENTS

URINARY TRACT STRUCTURE AND INFECTION

1

Chapter objectives

After studying this chapter you should be able to:

1. Describe the structure and embryological origins of the major anatomical components of the urinary tract, namely kidneys, ureters, bladder and urethra.

2. Understand the clinical distinction between upper and lower urinary tract infections.

3. Describe the organisms commonly associated with urinary infections and the mechanisms which make these organisms uropathogenic.

4. Describe the underlying factors associated with complicated urinary tract infections.

5. Select the most appropriate imaging techniques for the urinary tract when structural abnormalities are suspected.

6. Understand the principles of treatment of upper and lower urinary tract infections.

7. Describe the anatomical abnormalities and complications occurring in patients with vesicoureteric reflux.

Introduction

The kidneys are highly specialized organs that function to regulate the volume and chemical composition of the body fluids. In carrying out this function, they excrete most water-soluble waste products in urine. Once the urine is formed, it is collected and stored in the bladder. The bladder then empties intermittently during the process known as micturition.

When the normal processes of embryological development are disturbed, defects may develop in the structure of the urinary tract that interfere with the normal production and flow of urine. As a consequence, urinary tract infection may occur, and may be the initial clue that a structural abnormality of the urinary tract exists. This chapter, illustrated by the case of such an infection in a child, will introduce the basic structure and development of the kidneys and urinary tract, and discuss the common problem of urinary tract infection.

Normal anatomy of the urinary tract

The urinary tract is made up of the kidneys, ureters, bladder and urethra (Fig. 1.1). The kidneys are normally considered to be the upper urinary tract, whereas the remaining structures may be considered to be the lower urinary tract. There are normally two kidneys, each placed retroperitoneally in the posterior abdominal wall on either side of the spine at the level of the upper lumbar vertebrae. Each kidney is 10–14 cm in length in adults and is surrounded by a fibrous capsule within perirenal fat. The renal hilus on the concave medial aspect of the kidney is the point of entry for the arteries, veins and nerves, and exit for the urine drainage system. The urine formed by the kidney initially drains into the renal pelvis, which may be considered as the dilated portion of the ureter which links the kidney to the bladder. The urine in the renal pelvis is propelled by peristaltic action along the length of the ureter into the bladder. The ureters run medially and insert into the posterior base of the bladder, with the terminal end of the ureter tunnelled submucosally to form the vesicoureteric junction. The normal intrinsic musculature of the bladder surrounding the oblique course of the intravesical segment of the ureter is thought to be responsible for ureteric competence during bladder emptying, thus preventing the reflux of urine from the bladder back into the ureter. Abnormalities in the development of this intravesical segment are thought to predispose to the development of vesicoureteric reflux (see later in this chapter).

The bladder is an elastic organ consisting of connective tissue and smooth muscle, known as *detrusor*, loosely arranged in outer longitudinal, middle circular and inner longitudinal layers. This muscle arrangement results in the bladder's ability to empty during contraction. The dome of the bladder is covered by parietal peritoneum and is in apposition to other organs in the

---

Urinary tract structure and infection: 1

A febrile child

Tommy Baron is a 2-year-old boy who presents with a fever up to 39°C of 24 h duration. Although initially complaining of abdominal pain and unable to be comforted, he is now clearly ill, with lethargy and diffuse abdominal tenderness. His blood pressure is normal at 70/40 mm Hg. Examination is otherwise unremarkable. **Urinalysis** shows blood +++, protein ++ and is positive for leucocyte esterase (markers of white cells) and nitrites (markers of bacterial action).

We can infer from this information that Tommy is systemically unwell, with infection being the likely problem. The urinary abnormalities suggest the urinary tract is a source of the sepsis.

To understand the structural basis of this illness, we should initially familiarize ourselves with the anatomical components of the urinary tract. We can then consider whether Tommy is likely to have any abnormality that may predispose him to infection.

---

pelvis. The proximal urethra lies between the bladder neck and the pelvic diaphragm, and functionally consists of two sphincter mechanisms composed of both smooth and striated muscle. In women, the pelvic diaphragm is responsible for most of the sphincter mechanism. In men, the sphincter mechanism is largely incorporated into the prostate, with minimal sphincteric function incorporated into the bulbar and penile urethra.

Thus the kidneys and ureters are bilateral and paired, whereas the bladder and urethra are centrally placed and form a single structure. As a general principle, damage to a single kidney has minimal impact on overall renal excretory function provided the remaining kidney is normal. However, structural abnormalities of a single kidney or ureter may still predispose to infection, and may be relevant to Tommy's presentation, as will be discussed later in the chapter.

Structure of the kidney

The functional renal tissue, known as the renal parenchyma, is loosely divided into cortex and medulla. Each kidney contains about one million functional units, or nephrons, each consisting of a glomerulus and a tubule (Fig. 1.2). The glomerulus is responsible for filtering the blood, providing a barrier to the passage of protein and red blood cells into the urine. It is this filtrate which ultimately forms urine. After its production in the glomerulus, the filtrate enters the tubule, which functions to reabsorb and secrete fluid and electrolytes to adjust the urinary composition as necessary to maintain homeostasis of the body fluids. All nephrons have their glomeruli

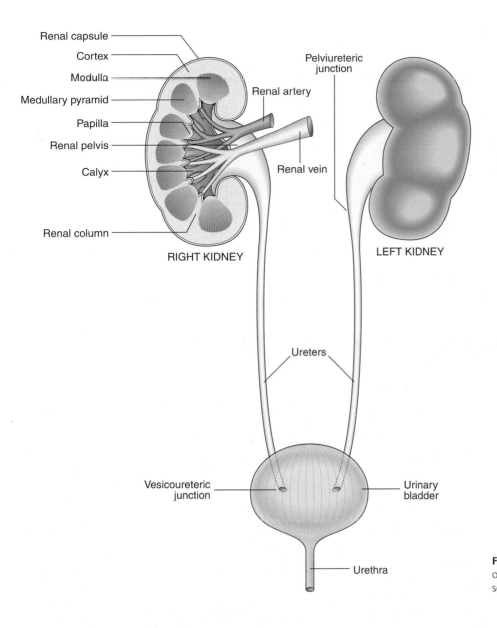

Renal capsule
Cortex
Modulla
Medullary pyramid
Papilla
Renal pelvis
Calyx
Renal column

Pelviureteric junction
Renal artery
Renal vein

RIGHT KIDNEY

LEFT KIDNEY

Ureters

Vesicoureteric junction

Urinary bladder

Urethra

Fig. 1.1 Principal anatomical components of the urinary tract, including features seen on a cut surface of the kidney.

located in the cortex, which comprises the outer one-third of the kidney. Approximately 15% of nephrons arise in the deepest part of the cortex (the juxtamedullary area). The inner two-thirds of the kidney consists of dark, striated areas known as pyramids, and the intervening renal columns, which together comprise the renal medulla. The apices of the pyramids are the renal papillae which project into the calyces, which are cuplike structures joining within the kidney to form the renal pelvis.

The glomerulus consists of a network of capillaries which invaginates the blinded end of the associated tubule, forming the Bowman's capsule. From this arises, in succession, the proximal tubule, the descending and ascending limbs of the loop of Henle, the distal tubule (including an early convoluted segment, a short connecting segment, and a late segment), the cortical collecting duct, the outer medullary and, subsequently, the inner medullary collecting duct, which opens at the tip of the

renal papilla into the renal pelvis. The structure and function of the renal tubular system and glomerulus are described in more detail in Chapters 2 and 5, respectively.

At least one renal artery supplies each kidney, but often multiple renal arteries are present. Each renal artery typically divides into five segments which subsequently branch up the sides of the pyramids, forming the interlobar arteries. At the junction of the medulla and cortex, the interlobar arteries divide into arcuate arteries. These then divide into interlobular arteries, giving rise to the afferent arterioles which feed into the glomeruli. The vessels emanating from the glomeruli are known as the efferent arterioles. The majority of efferent arterioles form a capillary network surrounding the proximal tubules within the cortex. However, the juxtamedullary glomeruli give rise to long, meshed capillary networks, the vasa recta, which participate in the countercurrent mechanism of urinary concentration in the kidney (see Chapter 3).

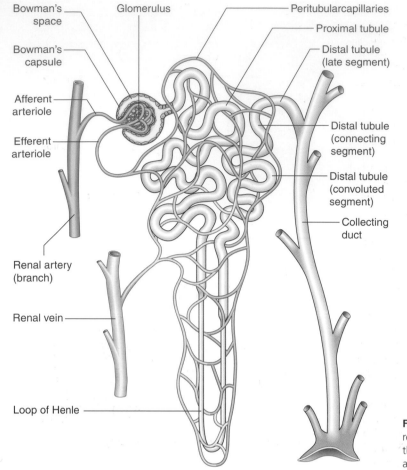

Bowman's space
Glomerulus
Peritubularcapillaries
Proximal tubule
Bowman's capsule
Distal tubule (late segment)
Afferent arteriole
Efferent arteriole
Distal tubule (connecting segment)
Distal tubule (convoluted segment)
Renal artery (branch)
Collecting duct
Renal vein
Loop of Henle

Fig. 1.2 Microscopic anatomy of the nephron showing relationship between vascular and tubular structures. Note that the anatomical arrangement of the juxtaglomerular apparatus is not illustrated here (see Chapter 2).

Innervation of the urinary tract

The neurological supply to the kidney is largely involved with regulation of vasomotor tone and hence renal blood flow. Sympathetic fibres originate in the lower splanchnic nerves and travel through the lumbar ganglion to the kidney. Stimulation of the sympathetic nervous system reduces renal blood flow by causing intrarenal vasoconstriction. It also enhances sodium reabsorption and stimulates the local renin–angiotensin system (see Chapter 2). However, denervated kidneys continue to function, usually without significant perturbations in major functional parameters.

Both sympathetic and parasympathetic nerve fibres supply the ureter. The spinal segments subtending this supply are the L1 and L2 nerve roots. Sympathetic fibres arising from the renal and intermesenteric plexuses supply the upper part of the ureter, the superior hypogastric plexus supplies the middle part, and the inferior hypogastric plexus (lying at the side of the bladder and prostate) supplies the lower part. Vagal fibres supply parasympathetic innervation to the kidney and ureter via the coeliac plexus and pelvic splanchnic nerves.

The bladder and urethra are innervated by both parasympathetic and sympathetic pathways. The parasympathetic fibres arise in the second to the fourth sacral nerve roots. They function to stimulate bladder emptying, vasodilatation and penile erection. The bladder is less densely innervated by sympathetic fibres which arise from T11–L3 nerve root segments. Stimulation of the sympathetic nervous system decreases bladder tone and inhibits the parasympathetic system. The base of the bladder and the proximal urethra are more richly innervated by sympathetic fibres which act to facilitate closure of the bladder neck and the proximal urethral sphincter. Drugs which block noradrenergic alpha-receptors (such as the antihypertensive prazosin) may inhibit periurethral sphincter function, resulting in incontinence. However these drugs are useful for relief of bladder outflow obstruction in benign prostatic hypertrophy, and for the relief of pain caused by ureteric spasm in the presence of an obstructing stone. The pelvic diaphragm is innervated by somatic motor neurones that allow voluntary contraction and relaxation. These neurones arise from the S2–S4 segments. The pelvic diaphragm is largely responsible for maintaining continence.

The bladder distends as urine is drained into it, resulting in the maintenance of low bladder pressures. This distension is essential to prevent urinary incontinence, which will occur if bladder pressures exceed the resistance of the urethral sphincter.

Micturition is therefore a complex process of coordinated stimulation of the parasympathetic nervous system which results in bladder contraction, and inhibition of sympathetic tone which results in sphincter relaxation. Voluntary control of voiding via the somatic nervous system is essential for regular drainage of the urinary tract to occur, as well as for social and hygiene reasons.

Embryology of the kidney and urinary tract

The development *in utero* of the urinary and reproductive tracts is closely related in both males and females. In the early stages of development, the urinary and genital ducts open into a common tract or cloaca, which is the dilated portion of the hindgut (see Fig. 1.3). In males, the urinary and genital systems continue to share a common distal excretory duct system, i.e. the distal urethra. However, in females the primitive excretory duct undergoes regression and does not form part of the reproductive tract in adults.

The fetus produces and excretes urine into the allantoic or amniotic fluid sac, where it is reabsorbed. The excretory function of the kidney is not essential until after delivery. However, if developmental anomalies of the urinary tract occur, they are often detected on fetal ultrasound because of the obstructed passage of urine.

Human kidneys are derived from the sequential development of the embryonic mesodermal kidney structures: the pronephros, mesonephros and metanephros. The pronephros degenerates in embryos of about 5 mm in length before full embryonic development. The mesonephros functions for a short time *in utero* as a provisional kidney before largely degenerating into the mesonephric tubule that persists to form part of the ductal system of the male reproductive tract. The metanephros remains and develops into the functional human kidney.

The excretory part of the metanephros develops from the portion of the nephrogenic cord caudal to the mesonephros. The functional human kidney is formed by invasion of the collecting tubules arising from the ureteric bud into the metanephric mesenchyme (Fig. 1.3). The branching and invasion of the ureteric bud into the mesenchyme is highly structured, showing several repeating patterns of division. As a result of this invasion, each tip of the branching collecting tubule has a 'cap' of approximately 100 mesenchymal cells, which are induced to survive, proliferate and undergo mesenchymal–epithelial transformation. These mesenchymal cells are effectively stem cells, capable of undergoing differentiation to form the glomeruli and the proximal loop and distal tubular segments of the nephron. This then joins the collecting tubule derived from the ureteric bud. In addition, the metanephric mesenchyme produces non-epithelial cells that are stromal in distribution. The cells of the mesenchyme and ureteric bud also produce factors which control the growth, differentiation and migration of endothelial, mesangial, smooth muscle and interstitial cells, as well as the deposition of extracellular matrix. These nephrons are

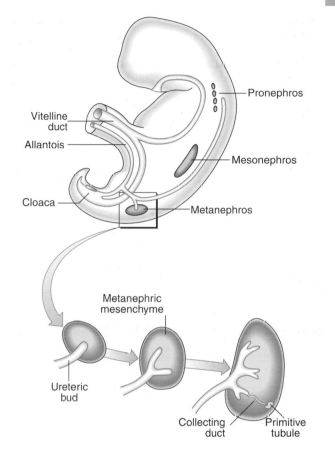

Fig. 1.3 Embryological development of the kidney.

grouped into lobules, which persist until birth and then generally disappear. However, some lobulation may persist into adult life.

During the development of the metanephros, the kidneys undergo an upward change in position, which is due partly to the cranial growth of the ureter and partly to the diminution of body curvature. Fusion of the lower poles of the kidney during this ascent results in the defect known as horseshoe kidney.

The impact that interference with the normal development of the kidney will have on the kidney and urinary tract depends on the stage of development at which the insult occurs. During the first few weeks of embryogenesis, an injury or insult may result in congenital absence of the kidney. If the same event occurs during the second or third month of gestation, parenchymal disruption may occur. This results in cystic or hypoplastic kidneys or abnormalities of the collecting systems, such as urethral atresia, posterior urethral valves or calyceal distortion. Vestigial tubules derived from metanephric tissue which fail to join the collecting ducts may result in closed secretory loops and form renal cysts. Early separation of the ureteric bud into two or more parts may result in duplex collecting systems. Beyond the fourth month of gestation, an insult is unlikely to affect the pelvicalyceal system, as it is well defined anatomically by this stage.

Case 1.1 Urinary tract structure and infection: 2

Tommy's test results

Tommy's blood tests demonstrated a high white cell count of 23.0×10^9/L* with a neutrophilia (increased neutrophil count) of 85%, suggestive of bacterial sepsis. The overall filtration function of his kidneys was normal, reflected by a serum creatinine concentration of 45 μmol/L. Blood and urine cultures were taken, and he was started on intravenous fluids and antibiotics. His urine culture subsequently demonstrated a pure growth of *E. coli*.

This information confirms the suspicion that Tommy has a urinary infection. We now need to consider the following issues.

1. Is it normal for microorganisms to be present in the urinary tract?
2. What are the factors that protect against organisms entering and infecting the urinary tract?
3. How is urinary tract infection diagnosed?

*Values are outside the normal range; see Appendix.

Table 1.1 Clinical features of acute lower and upper urinary tract infection in adults

Lower urinary tract infection	Upper urinary tract infection*
Dysuria	Systemically unwell
Frequency	Fever ± rigors
Suprapubic pain	Loin pain and tenderness
Malodorous urine	Nausea and vomiting
Haematuria	Hypotension or shock
Normal temperature	± Features of lower urinary tract infection

Acute infection of the upper urinary tract is also referred to as acute pyelonephritis.

The genetic and molecular basis of the processes that govern these regulated phases of renal embryonic development remain largely unknown. A number of genes, which produce a variety of molecules that may be potential regulators of renal development, have been identified. Disruption of these processes may result in a variety of developmental renal abnormalities.

One consequence of abnormal development of urinary tract structures may be impaired urinary drainage, and hence predisposition to infection. This possibility will be explored in relation to our febrile child.

Infection of the urinary tract

Infection of the urinary tract is one of the most common bacterial infections in both children and adults. The clinical features, diagnosis, treatment and significance of the infection vary depending on the site of infection and the presence or absence of structural and/or functional abnormalities within the urinary tract. Recurrent urinary infection, when complicated by major structural abnormalities, can lead to chronic kidney disease. In the presence of underlying kidney disease, superimposed infection often accelerates functional decline. However, recurrent uncomplicated urinary infection, although common and debilitating, generally has no long-term deleterious consequences.

Asymptomatic bacteriuria

Asymptomatic bacteriuria is defined as the presence of bacteria in the urinary tract in the absence of symptoms attributable to infection. Contamination of urine by organisms normally residing in the female periurethral area at the time of collection is common. Thus it is generally considered that 'significant bacteriuria' is present when 10^5 or more of the same organisms per millilitre are present in two voided urinary specimens (or in one 'in–out' catheter specimen) in a woman, or in one voided specimen in a man. In general, antibiotic treatment of asymptomatic bacteriuria is only indicated in the presence of factors leading to potentially complicated urinary infection (including pregnancy). In many circumstances, asymptomatic bacteriuria is a recurrent problem and antibiotic therapy may lead to antibiotic resistance that may cause infection to be more difficult to eradicate.

Acute urinary tract infection

Acute infection of the urinary tract can generally be divided on clinical grounds into upper or lower tract infection (Table 1.1).

The clinical presentation of urinary tract infection in children is much more variable and is frequently non-specific, as in Tommy's case. Thus children may present with lethargy, vomiting, fever, poor weight gain, irritability, febrile convulsions or gastrointestinal symptoms. Hence, the diagnosis should be considered in any sick infant or toddler.

Another basis of classification is whether the infection is 'complicated' (by systemic or anatomical abnormalities; Box 1.1) or 'uncomplicated'.

Lower urinary tract infections are particularly common in women, where they are generally localized to the bladder (cystitis). In adult men, the urethra and/or the prostate may be the primary site of infection. In the latter instances, sexually transmitted disease should be considered, particularly if no overt infection is isolated on urine culture (see below).

Upper urinary tract infection is defined as infection involving the kidney. As the renal pelvis is invariably

Box 1.1 Underlying factors associated with 'complicated' urinary tract infection

Systemic conditions

Diabetes mellitus
Papillary necrosis (e.g. analgesic nephropathy)
Immunodeficient states (including immunosuppressive drug therapy)

Abnormal drainage of urine

Renal calculi
Urinary obstruction
Vesicoureteric reflux
Pelviureteric junction obstruction
Instrumentation of the urinary tract (including catheters)

Pregnancy

Box 1.2 Microbiological agents causing urinary tract infection

Community-acquired

Escherichia coli
Klebsiella spp.
Proteus mirabilis
Staphylococcus saprophyticus

Hospital-acquired

Escherichia coli
Klebsiella spp.
Citrobacter spp.
Enterobacter spp.
Pseudomonas aeruginosa
Enterococcus faecalis

Coagulase-negative

Staphylococcus spp.
Candida spp. *

*These are yeasts (fungi).

involved in ascending infection, this is also referred to as acute pyelonephritis.

These arbitrary divisions have implications for treatment and prognosis, and guide decisions regarding further investigation. If the kidneys and urinary tract are normal anatomically and functionally, infection is unlikely to result in significant renal impairment, even when persistent and/or recurrent. However, if there is impaired renal function, reduced systemic resistance to infection, or abnormal drainage of the urinary tract, an infection is likely to become complicated, with the risk of renal damage, abscess formation or septicaemia. As dilatation and impaired drainage of the urinary tract is inevitable in pregnancy, all urinary infection in pregnant women should be treated as a potentially complicated infection (see also Chapter 11).

Aetiology and pathogenesis of urinary tract infection

There are numerous differences in the clinical features, response to therapy and prognosis of urinary infection according to the age of the patient, site of infection and whether the infection is complicated or uncomplicated. However, the microbial aetiology of infections is similar throughout the urinary system regardless of clinical setting.

Bacteria are by far the most common cause of urinary infection, with most other infecting organisms occurring in patients with underlying systemic illness (Box 1.2).

E. coli accounts for approximately 85% of community-acquired and 50% of hospital-acquired urinary infection. However, almost every organism has been associated with urinary tract infection, especially in the immuno-compromised inpatient population and in those with urological instrumentation. Organisms not traditionally regarded as urological pathogens may also occur in this population in whom natural host defence mechanisms are compromised. These organisms include lactobacilli, *Gardnerella vaginalis* and mycoplasma species, including *Ureaplasma urealyticum*. Staphylococcal pyelonephritis (almost always *S. aureus*) should always raise the possibility of haematogenous spread from distant foci as this is an unusual organism to colonize the periurethra and cause ascending infection.

Most episodes of urinary sepsis are caused by ascending infection, with a small percentage of upper urinary infections arising from the haematogenous (bloodborne) route. The vaginal introitus is normally colonized with a variety of non-virulent streptococci, staphylococci and lactobacilli, which are only occasionally responsible for urinary infection. Gram-negative bacteria, which are much more likely to cause urinary infection, normally reside in the bowel and colonize the introitus in a proportion of women. Factors thought to be responsible for periurethral colonization by colonic bacteria and subsequent bacterial entry into the bladder include previous antibiotic therapy, the use of a diaphragm and spermicide for contraceptive purposes, and sexual activity. In many instances an alteration in sexual activity (either sexual partner or frequency of intercourse) will predispose to urinary infection in women.

Different factors operate to prevent urinary infection at each anatomical level in the urinary tract. The common uropathogens are able to overcome the normal host defence mechanisms that protect against urinary infection. The relative contribution of bacterial virulence factors to infection depends on the site of infection as well as the normality or otherwise of the urinary tract. In the presence of an anatomically abnormal urinary tract, organisms of low virulence may still be able to establish a significant infection. However, this is rarely the case if such organisms infect a structurally normal urinary tract. Under normal circumstances bacteria introduced into the bladder are rapidly cleared by the constant urine flow, which serves to flush the bladder and dilute its contents. The direct antibacterial properties of the urine and of the bladder mucosa, as well as urinary constituents (such as high osmolarity, urea and organic acids), inhibit bacterial growth in the urine. However, the presence of glucose and amino acids may facilitate bacterial growth. Prostatic secretions have bactericidal properties, and white cells within the bladder mucosa participate in local defence against infection.

Bacterial virulence factors have been best studied in *E. coli* (Box 1.3), where a limited number of serotypes have been found to be responsible for the majority of infections. Various antigenic factors have been identified which enhance the urovirulence of a particular strain.

The adherence of *E. coli* to urothelial cells is predominantly determined by bacterial fimbriae, which are filamentous processes projecting from the cell surface. In addition, the capsules of *E. coli* contain specific virulence factors. Capsular antigens possess antiphagocytic activity and are important when tissue invasion occurs. As iron is a necessary bacterial nutrient, mechanisms to chelate and scavenge iron efficiently (siderophores) confer increased pathogenicity. Similarly, bacterial haemolysin production, which facilitates the release of haem, increases iron scavenging and thus virulence.

Urease production by organisms such as *Proteus mirabilis*, *P. vulgaris* and *S. saprophyticus* is involved in tissue adherence, and also in splitting urea into carbon dioxide and ammonia. This urease activity results in urinary alkalinization and precipitation of magnesium, ammonium and phosphate. Thus infection with these organisms often becomes complicated by stone formation (struvite).

Investigation of urinary tract infection

The laboratory diagnosis of urinary tract infection depends on microbiological confirmation of infection. This is usually taken to mean a bacterial count of greater than 10^5 colony-forming units (CFU) per millilitre. The technique of collection of the urine specimen is critical. In men the collection of a midstream specimen is usually successful and contamination is rare. In women, the introitus should be cleaned with saline (not antiseptic as this may inhibit bacterial growth and cause a falsely negative culture result). A midstream urine is collected with the labia spread apart. Collection in infants and children is difficult as adhesive bags are likely to become contaminated. In these circumstances suprapubic aspiration is a safe alternative that provides a definitive diagnosis. Urine can be stored at 4°C for up to 48 h before culture.

Although the laboratory cut-off for significant infection is regarded as 10^5 CFU/mL, infection may be present when colony counts are between 10^2 and 10^5 CFU/mL, particularly in the case of less common organisms such

Box 1.3 Virulence factors of uropathogenic *E. coli*

Lower urinary tract
Rapid growth rate
Adhesion to uroepithelial cells (bacterial fimbriae)
Endotoxin production (lipopolysaccharide)

Upper urinary tract
Resistance to serum bactericidal activity
Siderophore and haemolysin production
Resistance to phagocytosis
Persistence of organism within the kidney

as Gram-positive bacteria and some fungi. Mixed cultures, particularly in the presence of low colony counts in females, are usually the result of contamination.

Because of the delay inherent in microbiological confirmation of urinary tract infection, urinalysis is often used as a first line screen in individuals with symptoms suggestive of urinary infection (Fig. 1.4). Biochemical reagent strips will detect nitrites, which are produced by common uropathogens, and also leucocytes. The finding of pyuria (increased leucocyte excretion) does not always correlate with infection, since it may occur with other causes of urogenital inflammation and in normal pregnancy. Microscopic haematuria and proteinuria on urinalysis may be indicative of urinary tract inflammation, but are unreliable as markers of infection when additional renal or urinary tract pathology is present. Urine microscopy may demonstrate red cells, white cells and bacteria characteristic of infection. Evidence of white cell casts is suggestive of renal parenchymal infection. Additional tests have been developed to localize the site of infection to the upper or lower urinary tract, but these are not routinely used in clinical practice. In patients presenting with systemic features of pyelonephritis, septicaemia is possible and, in this clinical setting, blood should be taken for culture.

In otherwise healthy sexually active women, isolated lower urinary infection in the absence of systemic or structural factors predisposing to complicated infection (see Box 1.1) requires no further investigation, unless it is recurrent (more than three episodes per year). Urinary infection in males should be regarded as being potentially complicated, and underlying abnormalities of the urinary tract, particularly those causing obstruction of urine flow, should be sought. In younger males, congenital abnormalities of the urinary tract predominate, including vesicoureteric reflux and the presence of urethral valves, while in older males, bladder neck obstruction caused by prostatic hypertrophy or urethral stricture is more likely. In appropriate male patients, it is important also to exclude active prostatitis or sexually transmitted disease. Further imaging investigations are necessary in cases where structural abnormality in the urinary tract

Fig. 1.4 Patterns of investigation in urinary tract infection. UTI, urinary tract infection; STDs, sexually transmitted diseases; MCU, micturating cystourethrogram.

Urinary tract structure and infection: 3

The next step

The severity of the systemic features in Tommy's case suggest that an underlying abnormality of the urinary tract may account for the infection. Indeed, the above discussion would suggest that, if free drainage of the urinary tract existed, infection is unlikely to have taken hold, particularly in a male.

In light of Tommy's age, the most likely underlying cause is a congenital abnormality of the urinary tract. In an older person, acquired abnormalities of the urinary tract are more commonly found. The nature of the structural abnormality is often easily determined by simple imaging of the urinary tract. This raises the issue of what techniques are available to gain a view of the anatomy of the urinary tract in different clinical settings.

---

is suspected, as in any child with UTI, or any patient with complicated or upper urinary tract infection.

Imaging of the urinary tract

Renal ultrasound is the initial screening test used for imaging the urinary tract in children, in men, or in the presence of complicated infection. It will define whether urinary tract dilatation is present and whether the underlying renal size and parenchymal thickness is normal (Fig. 1.5). The level of obstruction is suggested but the result may not be definitive, and computed tomography (CT scanning) may be indicated subsequently (Fig. 1.6). CT is rarely indicated in the acute setting of infection, but is frequently performed as a follow-up investigation especially where resolution is slow or incomplete. CT is also the best imaging modality if abscess formation is suspected, both to define the intrarenal mass as well as to monitor the response to therapy.

Intravenous pyelography (IVP) provides a functional and anatomical assessment of drainage of the urinary tract, particularly after correction of obstructive pathology or in the investigation of pelvicalyceal disease (see Fig. 1.9). However, it is now less commonly undertaken, and has largely been superseded by CT scanning and magnetic resonance imaging (see Table 12.2) where these newer modalities are available.

A radionuclide blood flow scan is of use in assessing renal perfusion (see Chapter 10) and avoids exposure to potentially nephrotoxic contrast agents.

Cystoscopy (direct inspection of the interior of the bladder) should be performed if primary bladder or prostate pathology is suspected. It is rarely indicated in patients with urinary infection who have normal upper tracts demonstrated on ultrasound. If impaired bladder function is suspected, urodynamic studies which record changes in pressure during bladder filling and emptying may be indicated.

All children presenting with urinary infection should be investigated with imaging of the urinary tract since up to 50% will be found to have a urological abnormality. In the majority of these children, vesicoureteric reflux

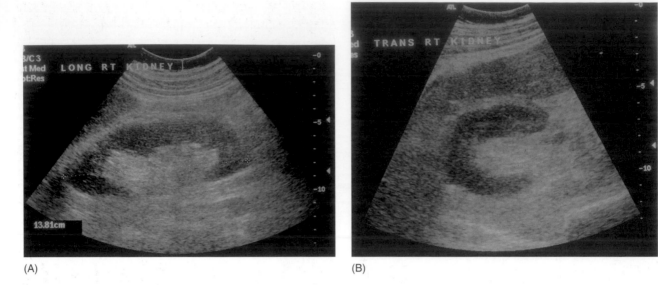

(A) (B)

Fig. 1.5 Normal renal ultrasound (long axis (A) and transverse axis (B) views).

(A) (B)

Fig. 1.6 CT scan of normal kidneys, in coronal (A) and axial (B) views. Corticomedullary differentiation is enhanced as a result of injection of contrast agent.

(see Box 1.4) will be confirmed. In infants who are acutely unwell with pyelonephritis, both ultrasound and micturating cystourethrogram (MCU) should be performed. The MCU demonstrates the presence of backflow of urine from the bladder into the ureters during micturition (vesicoureteric reflux). In older children an MCU is not always considered necessary in the presence of a good quality ultrasound view of the upper urinary tract, with visualization of the ureteric orifices and ureteric peristalsis. A radionuclide scan using DMSA (dimercaptosuccinic acid) is performed to detect renal parenchymal scarring (Fig. 1.7). This is not generally undertaken within 6–12 months of acute pyelonephritis to avoid false positive results.

Vesicoureteric reflux

Vesicoureteric reflux (VUR) is caused by incompetence of the vesicoureteric junction. In most instances the defect is one of shortness of the submucosal segment because of

(A)   (B)

Fig. 1.7 (A) Normal dimercaptosuccinic acid (DMSA) renal scan; (B) DMSA renal scan showing multiple cortical defects and severe bilateral renal scarring, worse in the upper pole.

Box 1.4 Features of vesicoureteric reflux and reflux nephropathy

---

Vesicoureteric reflux

Ultrasound *in utero* (incidental finding)
Enuresis
Double voiding
Loin pain on micturition
Urinary tract infection
Family screening

Reflux nephropathy

Hypertension
Proteinuria
Renal impairment
Impaired urine concentration *with or without features of VUR*

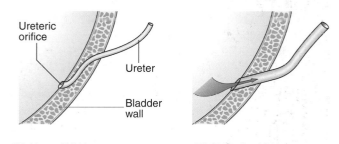

(A) Normal VUJ   **(B)** Refluxing VUJ

Fig. 1.8 Vesicoureteric junction (VUJ): (A) normal; (B) defective, with reflux.

lateral ectopia (displacement) of the ureteric orifice. This results in loss of the normal valvelike action associated with the oblique path of the terminal segment of ureter through the bladder wall (Fig. 1.8).

In the majority of infants, VUR presents with a complicating urinary infection. However, signs localizing the infection to the urinary tract may not always be present, especially in the very young. In males particularly, infection may not always occur, and more subtle signs of renal damage caused by retrograde urine flow (reflux nephropathy) may be present (Box 1.4).

If enuresis (bed-wetting) persists until after primary school age (10 years), reflux should be excluded with renal ultrasonography. Enuresis in this setting is caused by the presence of residual urine after voiding as the upper urinary tract empties into the bladder, and also by impaired tubular function with loss of the ability to concentrate the urine which leads to increased urine volumes. In adults, enuresis rarely persists but nocturia may be a prominent symptom.

It has recently been recognized that reflux nephropathy is inherited as an autosomal dominant condition. Thus current recommendations advise routine ultrasound in neonates of parents known to have reflux nephropathy independent of the grade of reflux in the affected parent. Recent research also suggests that a small and scarred kidney may be the primary congenital abnormality in at least some cases, with abnormalities of the vesicoureteric junction an associated or secondary development.

The diagnosis of VUR is based on demonstration of reflux on an MCU or real time ultrasound. There may also be radiological findings of focal scarring in the

Diagnosis and management

Soon after admission, Tommy underwent renal ultrasonography, which showed that the right kidney was 2 cm smaller than the left, with generalized loss of cortical thickness. The pelvis and ureter were dilated down to the level of the vesicoureteric junction but no obstruction was demonstrated. The right ureteric insertion into the bladder was laterally placed, and ureteric 'jets' (indicating normal pulsatile flow of urine from the ureter to the bladder) were not seen. This was taken as evidence of an abnormality of the vesicoureteric junction on that side. No abnormality was observed in the left kidney, pelvis or collecting system, and a normal left ureteric insertion and ureteric jets were noted.

After starting antibiotics (ceftriaxone), Tommy became afebrile with improved appetite over the ensuing 72 h. Intravenous antibiotics were continued for a total of 7 days, after which he was given oral cefaclor for a further week. Tommy was subsequently maintained on a preventative dose of trimethoprim/sulfamethoxazole at night. A repeat urine culture 3 weeks after his initial presentation was sterile.

It was recommended that his two siblings, aged 5 and 7 years, who were asymptomatic, should undergo screening urine culture and ultrasonography for the detection of vesicoureteric reflux.

It is clear that an underlying anatomical abnormality has contributed to Tommy's infection. Vesicoureteric reflux is one of the commonest congenital abnormalities of the urogenital tract. The following questions are likely to be raised by Tommy's parents and will be discussed:

1. What causes vesicoureteric reflux?
2. How is it diagnosed?
3. What treatment is indicated?

Fig. 1.9 Intravenous pyelogram showing gross scarring of left kidney, with clubbing of calyces characteristic of reflux nephropathy. Normal right kidney and collecting system.

renal parenchymal scarring is present, even in unilateral reflux, antireflux surgery does not protect against progressive decline in renal function.

Overall, reflux nephropathy accounts for approximately 5–8% of patients with end-stage renal failure in Australia and New Zealand, and 20–25% of the paediatric population with end-stage renal failure. Reflux nephropathy with progressive functional deterioration is characterized by hypertension and persistent proteinuria, which is a poor prognostic feature.

Overview: treatment of urinary tract infections

Most episodes of uncomplicated lower urinary tract infection are isolated events affecting sexually active women. Suitable antibiotics for use in this setting include trimethoprim, cefalexin and amoxicillin/clavulanate. In most cases, a 3-day course of therapy provides adequate treatment. In relapsing infection, a 10–14-day course of antibiotics should be prescribed and if infection persists or recurs investigation should be undertaken. Recurrent infection (more than three episodes per year) is best treated with prophylactic low-dose antibiotics. However, in patients with a clear relation between infection and sexual activity, single dose therapy after intercourse may be effective. Generally, follow-up cultures are not needed in otherwise uncomplicated urinary infection.

The treatment of acute upper urinary tract infection (acute pyelonephritis) is generally performed in hospital. Intravenous fluids and empiric antibiotic treatment (e.g. intravenous third generation cephalosporin such as ceftriaxone, with or without an aminoglycoside such as gentamicin) should be commenced before culture results

kidneys, generally at the upper pole, with calyceal clubbing. If more severe VUR is present, the kidney may be diffusely damaged with generalized loss of parenchymal tissue (Fig. 1.9).

VUR is the commonest underlying cause of hypertension in children and is associated with the presence of renal scarring. VUR may present in adults with moderate to severe hypertension without a history of urinary infection. Renal calculi are commonly present in areas of scarring within the kidney and presumably relate to urinary stasis. Urinary infection with *P. mirabilis* or other urea-splitting organisms may be associated with staghorn calculi but, with appropriate early treatment of infection with antibiotics, this is a relatively rare complication.

Antireflux surgery to correct the incompetence of the vesicoureteric junction is not generally recommended unless severe reflux causing upper tract dilatation is present. Corrective surgery is not undertaken after 2–3 years of age. It has long been appreciated that once

Urinary tract structure and infection: 5

Follow-up

At review 12 months later, Tommy's urine remains sterile with no proteinuria, and his growth and milestones appear normal. His blood pressure is at the upper limit of normal at 90/60 mm Hg. Repeat renal ultrasound is unchanged from that performed during the acute phase of his illness, although the right renal parenchyma is now less oedematous and the kidney measures 2.5 cm smaller than the left. A DMSA scan is performed which shows diffuse parenchymal cortical scars on the right, but none in the left kidney.

The management plan for Tommy is to maintain the prophylactic antibiotic until he is 5 years of age, and then repeat the ultrasound and DMSA scan. In the absence of new scar formation, it is planned that antibiotics will be ceased at that stage. Regular follow-up of blood pressure and urinalyses are advised to detect any increase in urinary protein excretion.

His 7-year-old sister has sterile urine, but renal ultrasonography and subsequent DMSA scan are suggestive of a right upper pole scar. There is no ultrasound evidence of ongoing reflux, with ureteric peristalsis and ureteric jets appearing normal. The management plan is to have 6-monthly urinalyses and a repeat DMSA scan in 1 year. In the absence of infection and progressive renal scarring, her blood pressure and urinalysis will be monitored on a 2–3-yearly basis. The risks of infection in pregnancy and potential for developing hypertension, particularly in pregnancy, are explained to her mother for future information. The remaining sibling is normal.

become available. An appropriate oral antibiotic with good renal parenchymal penetration, such as amoxicillin/clavulanate or norfloxacin, may be substituted when the fever subsides. The total duration of antibiotic treatment is generally 2 weeks. If no significant improvement is observed within 48h, the diagnosis and choice of antibiotic therapy should be reviewed, and imaging of the kidney undertaken to exclude obstruction or abscess.

BODY FLUIDS, NEPHRON FUNCTION AND DIURETICS

Chapter objectives

After studying this chapter you should be able to:

1. Describe the normal distribution and composition of body fluids.

2. Give some causes and clinical features of hypovolaemia and hypervolaemia.

3. Describe the functional anatomy of the nephron.

4. Give an account of the main sodium transport processes in the nephron, and the normal regulation of sodium and potassium excretion.

5. Describe the site and mechanism of action of commonly used diuretic drugs.

6. Outline some common disturbances of sodium and potassium balance.

Introduction

The main function of the kidney is not 'to produce urine' (this is an inconvenient byproduct rather than a biological necessity), but to regulate the volume and composition of the body fluids within narrow limits. While the best known task performed by the kidney is filtration of the blood, this is really just the first step in a sequence of actions whereby the functional unit of the kidney, the nephron, responds to disturbances in the volume and composition of the circulating fluids. This results in the excretion of urine as a byproduct.

While many types of kidney disease can interfere with these processes, significant alterations in nephron function can be produced even in a person with normal kidneys by pharmacological agents which interfere with the normal physiological mechanisms operating in the nephron. As illustrated by the case discussed in this chapter, this can have serious implications for the volume and electrolyte composition of the plasma. See Case 2.1:1.

Body fluid and electrolyte distribution

A number of features of Joanne's history and physical examination suggest that her total body fluid volume is reduced. First, her symptoms of light-headedness and near-fainting attacks suggest that her cardiovascular system is unable to maintain perfusion of her brain, especially when she is upright. This inference is confirmed on physical examination, where it is found that she has a lowish lying blood pressure which falls further on standing, accompanied by a marked increase in her pulse rate. These features are suggestive of activated sympathetic nervous system responses to maintain her cardiac output in the face of a low circulating fluid volume. Her dry mouth and flaccid skin are suggestive of depletion of mucosal and tissue water, consistent with dehydration.

A summary of clinical features of hypovolaemia (sometimes loosely called dehydration, which strictly refers to a pure water deficit) contrasted with features typically found in hypervolaemia (also called fluid overload) is given in Table 2.1. As will be explained further below, these disturbances come about more through underlying disturbances of body sodium content than from primary changes in body water.

Since we suspect that something has depleted Joanne's body of fluid, we need to ask this question: how is water normally distributed within the body, and what is the composition of the fluid in different body compartments?

Body fluid compartments

The total body water content for a typical adult is approximately 60% of the lean body mass, i.e. about 40 litres in

---

Body fluids and nephron function: 1

Fluid and electrolyte depletion

Joanne Smithfield is a 19-year-old woman who presents to her family doctor complaining of weakness and light-headedness. These symptoms have been troubling her for some 6 months, but in the last week she has become more concerned as she has had a number of near-fainting episodes at work. These attacks are usually initiated by getting up rapidly from her desk, which makes her feel light-headed until she sits or lies down again. She has also noticed increasing difficulty walking up the stairs in her block of flats, where she lives with a girlfriend on the second floor. She attributes this to weakness in her legs, though she had previously been a strong runner at school.

Joanne's past medical history is unremarkable. Her menarche (commencement of menstruation) was at age 11 years, and her periods have been regular in timing and moderate in volume. She mentioned that she had gained too much weight as an adolescent, but considered that this was now 'under control'. Her family history includes hypertension and heart failure diagnosed recently in her father, but her mother is well at age 48 years and is a fitness instructor. She has a younger sister who is a keen athlete. Joanne smokes 10 cigarettes/day and drinks a little alcohol after work on some days and on weekends. Her only medications are occasional laxatives when she gets constipated, and 'fluid tablets' to remove puffiness around her ankles which she thinks makes her look unattractive.

On physical examination, Joanne looks well though a little tired. She takes a few moments to stand up from her chair, and steadies herself against the wall after doing so. Her tongue and mouth appear rather dry, and her skin feels quite doughy. Her blood pressure is 105/70 lying, 95/70 sitting, 85/65 standing. The pulse rate increases from 85 beats/min lying to 105 beats/min standing. Heart sounds are normal, and the lung fields are clear. Abdominal examination is unremarkable, although some stretch marks are noted. Neurological examination reveals normal cranial nerves, but moderate weakness proximally in the upper and lower limbs. Reflexes and sensory testing are normal.

At the end of the examination, Joanne is questioned further about her use of diuretic tablets. She confesses that lately she has been taking one or two furosemide (frusemide; Lasix) tablets daily, as she finds this helps to keep her weight down and avoid swelling around her ankles and hips. She initially obtained these from her father, but subsequently got them from a friend who is prescribed them by her family doctor for premenstrual swelling.

In response to this presentation we can ask the questions:

1. What physiological disturbances are causing Joanne's symptoms?
2. How might these disturbances have come about?

Table 2.1	Clinical features of hypovolaemia and hypervolaemia	
	Hypovolaemia	*Hypervolaemia*
Symptoms	Thirst	Ankle swelling
	Dizziness on standing	Breathlessness
	Weakness	Abdominal swelling
Signs	Low JVP	Oedema
	Postural hypotension	Raised JVP
	Tachycardia	Pulmonary crepitations
	Dry mouth	Pleural effusion
	Reduced skin turgor	Ascites
	Reduced urine output	Hypertension
	Weight loss	(sometimes)
	Confusion, stupor	Weight gain
JVP, jugular venous pressure.		

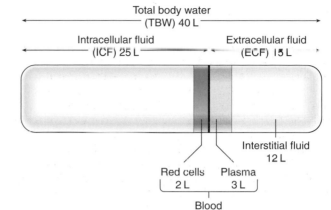

Fig. 2.1 Compartments of distribution of total body water. Approximate volumes (in litres) are shown for an average adult.

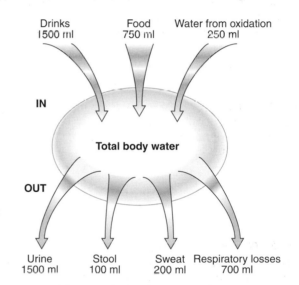

Fig. 2.2 Typical fluxes involved in daily water balance.

an average 70 kg man. This can be determined by studying the dilution of marker substances which are known to distribute into all compartments of the body water.

The most familiar fraction of body fluid, namely the blood, represents a relatively small compartment of the total body water. Indeed, Fig. 2.1 shows that some 62.5% (5/8ths) of the total body water is actually located inside cells (the intracellular fluid or ICF), while 37.5% (3/8ths) is in the extracellular fluid compartment (ECF). Furthermore, the plasma component of the blood accounts for a relatively small part (around 20%) of the ECF, with the remainder being distributed as interstitial fluid (ISF) within the various organs and tissues of the body but outside the cells. It can also be seen from Fig. 2.1 that the blood is actually composed in part of ECF (the plasma component) and in part ICF (the red cells).

In a normal individual, the volumes in the various body fluid compartments are remarkably constant in the face of somewhat variable water intake from one day to another. This constancy, an example of the *homeostasis* of the body's internal environment, is dependent on a number of finely tuned regulatory mechanisms which will be outlined in this and the next chapter, and in other books in this series. In brief, a state of equilibrium (or balance) is achieved such that the net intake of water, largely by mouth under normal circumstances, is matched by the total losses through the skin, lungs, gut and kidneys. Typical volumes involved in these fluxes on a daily basis are shown in Fig. 2.2. It is important to understand that the major control mechanism for adjusting water loss from the body to match daily water intake resides in the kidney. The kidney has a highly regulated capacity to vary the daily output of urine, while losses from the other sites are largely fixed.

Body fluid composition

There are important differences in the solute composition of the various compartments of body fluid, and these have major implications for normal cell metabolism, and

for the normal function of the circulatory and neuromuscular systems.

The major features of the chemical make-up of the ICF and the ECF (the latter having two major subdivisions, the plasma and the interstitial fluid) are shown in Fig. 2.3.

In brief, the main distinction between the ICF and the ECF is that the dominant cation in the ECF is sodium (Na^+) while in the ICF it is potassium (K^+). Chloride and bicarbonate make up most of the balancing anions in the ECF, while in the ICF the principal negative charges are carried by phosphate and other organic anions. In addition, there is an important contribution to the intracellular anion pool from negative charges on the many cellular proteins contained in that compartment. There is normally a zero net flux of water across the cell membrane, i.e. the ECF and ICF are in 'osmotic equilibrium'.

The mechanism for establishing and maintaining this substantial gradient for cations between the interior and exterior of cells is the membrane-bound sodium–potassium 'pump' (Na,K-activated ATPase). This ubiquitous active transport carrier uses energy derived directly

Fig. 2.3 Chemical composition of different compartments of body water. ICF, intracellular fluid; ECF, extracellular fluid.

from the hydrolysis of ATP to extrude three sodium ions from the cell for every two potassium ions it takes up from the ECF. The pump itself is thus 'electrogenic' and contributes towards generating the inside-negative membrane potential of the cell. A more significant contribution, however, comes from the back-diffusion of intracellular potassium ions to the cell exterior through potassium channels present in the cell membrane.

The significance of the gradient for Na and K maintained across cell membranes in all body tissues is profound. First, high intracellular K concentrations are essential for the normal operation of many enzyme systems which drive cell metabolism. Second, the basis of electrical excitability of neuromuscular and cardiac membranes is the presence of steep concentration gradients for Na and K across these membranes. Third, the capacity of epithelia which line interfaces between the body and the exterior to carry out net transepithelial solute transport depends on the maintenance of Na and K gradients in cells of these tissues. In the last case, however, the pump units are asymmetrically distributed in opposing cell membrane surfaces (illustrated for the kidney later in this chapter).

Another important distinction is that existing between the composition of the plasma and ISF components of the ECF. As shown in Fig. 2.3, the main difference here is that the plasma, but not the ISF, contains a substantial concentration of proteins, comprising both serum albumin as well as a spectrum of globulins.

The mechanism for maintaining this protein differential within the subsections of the ECF is the presence of a permeability barrier at the capillary wall which largely prevents the movement of proteins out of the capillaries under normal circumstances.

The significance of this protein concentration gradient is that it makes an important contribution to the balance of forces across the capillary wall (specifically to the colloid osmotic – or oncotic – pressure of the plasma), favouring fluid retention within the capillaries, thus maintaining an adequate circulating plasma volume. The effect of disturbance of this gradient will be illustrated in the discussion of oedema states in Chapter 6 of this volume.

The central importance of sodium for stability of the circulation

From the above discussion it is clear that sodium is the dominant ionic species in the ECF since, together with its accompanying anions, it accounts for over 95% of the

Box 2.1 Causes of hypovolaemia and hypervolaemia

Hypovolaemia

- **Gastrointestinal sodium loss**
  e.g. vomiting, diarrhoea, nasogastric suction
- **Skin sodium loss**
  e.g. excessive sweating, burns
- **Renal sodium loss**
  e.g. diuretics, mineralocorticoid deficiency, tubulointerstitial disease
- **Internal sequestration**
  e.g. bowel obstruction, peritonitis, pancreatitis, crush injury
- **Haemorrhage**

Hypervolaemia

- **Iatrogenic**
  e.g. salt loading (oral or intravenous)
- **Renal sodium retention in generalized oedema states**
  e.g. congestive cardiac failure, cirrhosis, nephrotic syndrome
- **Renal sodium retention in renal failure**
  e.g. acute and chronic kidney disease (usual case)
- **Renal sodium retention in primary mineralocorticoid excess**
  e.g. Conn's syndrome (note no oedema)

Case 2.1 Body fluids and nephron function: 2

A probable culprit

So far we can deduce from the cardiovascular clues in the history and physical examination that Joanne has probably experienced a reduction in the circulating component of the ECF, namely the plasma. The dryness of her mouth and laxity of her skin suggest that other tissue fluid compartments are also depleted of water.

While a number of causes for this situation may be considered, in this case we have the information that she has been taking a drug which is intended to cause the kidneys to excrete higher than normal volumes of urine, causing her total body water content to be reduced.

A number of new questions now arise related to the role of the kidney in the origin of Joanne's problem, namely:

1. How does the kidney normally make urine?
2. How has the diuretic drug interfered with these processes to lead to body fluid depletion?

solute present in this fluid compartment. This is equivalent to saying that sodium is responsible for nearly all of the osmotic activity in the ECF (the 'oncotic' pressure attributable to plasma proteins, referred to above, is much smaller, though it is important as a differential osmotic force across capillary membranes). Thus, when water is added to the body, the amount held in the ECF is largely determined by the body's sodium content, since the great majority of sodium ions are confined to the ECF compartment.

This gives rise to the important clinical deduction that factors which deplete the body of sodium will be associated with a low ECF volume (and hence of circulating plasma), while sodium retention is associated with expanded ECF volume. A summary of the causes of hypovolaemia and hypervolaemia based on sodium disturbances is given in Box 2.1. Note that pure disturbances in body mechanisms for regulating water itself are relatively uncommon causes of these conditions, but are more likely to produce changes in plasma sodium concentration and osmolality (see Chapter 3).

Functional anatomy of the nephron

In fundamental terms, the kidney provides a site of interface between the circulating blood and the outside world.

At this interface, a number of regulatory processes occur which allow for a finely tuned response by the kidney to signals concerning the volume and composition of the circulating plasma, leading to the excretion from the body of urine whose volume and composition represent a byproduct of these processes.

The functional unit in which these interchanges are carried out within the kidney is the nephron. It is a microscopic structure consisting of a glomerulus, or 'small ball' of capillaries derived from the renal arterial supply, closely associated with an elongated tubelike structure (the tubular system) which is lined by a single layer of epithelial cells.

As shown schematically in Fig. 2.4, the two fundamental steps in nephron function are glomerular filtration, and modification of the filtered fluid as it passes through the tubular system.

Glomerular filtration

Glomerular filtration is the process whereby a clear fluid, from which blood cells and macromolecules such as proteins are excluded, is produced from the blood perfusing the glomerulus at the beginning of each nephron. This ultrafiltration process, which occurs largely as a result of the hydrostatic pressure in the arterial tree generated by the heart, is described in more detail in Chapter 5. The ultrafiltrate so produced contains electrolytes and small solutes in plasma-like concentrations, and constitutes the 'primary' urine from which the final excreted urine is derived.

Fig. 2.4 Functional anatomy of the nephron.

Tubular modification

This step involves the alteration of the volume and composition of the glomerular filtrate by transport processes carried out along the length of the tubular system. The dominant modification overall is the reabsorption of the great majority (over 99%) of the filtered fluid, together with most of its solute content (notably sodium). However, some electrolytes and many 'foreign' organic molecules undergo transport *into* the tubular fluid, a process called secretion. The final urine excreted from the kidneys reflects the net effect of all these tubular transport processes.

It is important to note in Fig. 2.4 that not all of the blood plasma brought to the nephron is filtered at the glomerulus. Of the plasma flow delivered to each nephron, some 20% becomes glomerular filtrate while the remaining 80% emerges from the glomerulus and is carried by postglomerular capillaries around the tubular structures of that (and adjacent) nephrons, where it is available for transport exchanges with the luminal fluid. The ratio of the glomerular filtration rate (GFR) to the renal plasma flow (RPF) is called the filtration fraction (FF), and is about 0.2 in man.

Some approximate figures will serve to illustrate the relative magnitude of these processes. The kidneys receive about one-fifth of the cardiac output, which for an adult woman like Joanne may be 4.5 L/min. Thus the total renal blood flow (RBF) would be 900 mL/min. Assuming a haematocrit (red blood cell volume as a fraction of total blood volume) of 0.45, the RPF would be almost 500 mL/min (i.e. $(1 - 0.45) \times 900$). If the filtration fraction is 0.2, her GFR will be 100 mL/min. Given 99% reabsorption of the filtrate volume, this corresponds to a typical urine flow rate of 1 mL/min. On a daily basis, the corresponding figures are a GFR of 144 litres/24h, and a daily urine output of 1.4 litres/24h.

Nephron segments

A more anatomically detailed view of the tubular structures comprising the nephron is given in Fig. 2.5. Each of the kidney's one million nephrons has its glomerulus

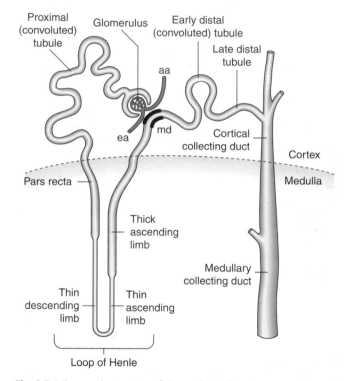

Fig. 2.5 Microscopic structure of the nephron, showing names of successive tubular segments. aa, afferent arteriole; ea, efferent arteriole; md, macula densa. (Refer to Fig. 1.2 for details of vascular elements.)

located in the renal cortex (see Chapter 1). Blood is delivered through a series of branches of the renal artery until it enters each glomerulus via an afferent arteriole. After breaking up into the capillary loops constituting the glomerulus, the blood emerges via an efferent arteriole which itself gives rise to the network of peritubular capillaries. These eventually join to take the blood away from the kidney via the renal vein. (The vascular structures are shown in more detail in Fig. 1.2.)

The segments of the tubular system attached to each glomerulus are named, in order, the proximal tubule, the loop of Henle, the distal tubule and the collecting duct. Each segment consists of specialized epithelial cells adapted to perform particular transport functions.

The proximal tubule is some 2–3 mm long. It forms a number of turns, or convolutions, before descending in a straight segment (pars recta) down into the outer medulla. Its cells are characterized by a prominent brush border consisting of numerous elongated processes arising from the apical (lumen-facing) cell membrane. Many mitochondria lie between the extensive invaginations of the basolateral (blood-facing) membrane.

The loop of Henle descends from the outer medulla a variable distance into the inner medulla, going deepest for loops arising from nephrons having their glomeruli located in the inner cortex (the juxtamedullary nephrons). It consists of a thin descending limb and, after a hairpin turn, a shorter thin ascending segment, both of which comprise flat cells with few mitochondria and little membrane amplification. The cells of the thick ascending limb, on the other hand, are larger and contain abundant mitochondria and extensive basolateral infoldings, suggestive of a role in active ion transport.

The distal tubule starts within the cortex at the point where the thick ascending limb passes by the glomerulus of the related nephron, where it forms the macula densa (see later in this chapter). The early part of the distal tubule is convoluted, with metabolically active cells. After a short connecting segment, the late distal tubule is straight, and joins with similar segments from adjacent nephrons to form the cortical collecting duct, with which it has structural and functional similarities (and indeed a common embryological origin from the ureteric bud; see Fig. 1.3).

The medullary collecting duct arises in continuity with the cortical collecting duct as it crosses the corticomedullary junction. The lumen becomes progressively wider as it passes towards the tip of the renal papilla, where it empties into the calyces and the renal pelvis.

Sodium transport

An appreciation of the mechanisms involved in handling sodium in the nephron is of crucial importance in understanding how our patient's body fluid depletion has come about. As mentioned previously, over 99% of the fluid filtered is normally reabsorbed along the tubular system of the nephron, and this is largely related to the reabsorption of a similar proportion of filtered sodium. Assuming a plasma Na concentration of 140 mmol/L and a GFR of 144 L/day, the amount of sodium passed into the filtrate is 140×144, which equals 20,160 mmol/day. For a person consuming some 100 mmol of sodium per day in the diet, daily balance with regard to sodium requires the excretion of 100 mmol Na/day into the final urine (neglecting the very small losses through the gut and skin). This represents just (100/20,160) or 0.5% of the sodium contained in the glomerular filtrate, so we conclude that 99.5% of the filtered sodium load must be reabsorbed by the tubules.

The segments in which this reabsorptive activity occurs have been defined by micropuncture experiments

Table 2.2 Sodium reabsorption in successive segments of the nephron

Tubular segment	Sodium reabsorption
Proximal tubule	65%
Loop of Henle (thick ascending limb)	25%
Distal tubule	
Early (convoluted segment)	6%
Late (initial/cortical collecting duct)	2–3%
Medullary collecting duct	<1%

Amounts reabsorbed at each site are expressed as a percentage of the filtered load of sodium.

in animal models. Microscopic amounts of fluid are sampled from different points along the nephron, and their composition is compared to that of the filtered fluid. Table 2.2 shows the estimated contributions by successive tubular segments under normal conditions which have been deduced by these experiments.

In the following sections, an outline of the cellular mechanism of sodium reabsorption in each of these segments will be provided.

Proximal tubule

Much of the cortical tissue mass in the kidney consists of proximal tubules, and these are the most metabolically active cells in the kidney. This activity is directed primarily towards the reabsorption of some two-thirds (nearly 70%) of the sodium contained in the glomerular filtrate, together with associated solutes and water.

The mechanisms involved in this reabsorptive process are complex, and will only be outlined here. The following are some transport properties of the proximal tubule:

- The process occurs almost isotonically, i.e. the osmolality of the tubular fluid falls only very slightly below that of the plasma along the length of the tubule.

- Sodium reabsorption is associated with complete reabsorption of filtered glucose and amino acids (when plasma concentrations are normal), and almost complete reabsorption of bicarbonate and phosphate ions.

- Reabsorption of all solutes and water is very sensitive to metabolic poisons.

- There is a very high water permeability across the proximal tubular cell layer.

- There is a low electrical potential difference across the tubular epithelial wall.

From these and other detailed observations, a model for the operation of a typical cell in this tubular segment has been developed, as shown in Fig. 2.6.

The primary active transport step underlying absorption of sodium and, secondarily, other solutes and water,

Fig. 2.6 Principal transport properties of a proximal tubule cell. Open circles represent carrier molecules without direct linkage to ATP hydrolysis; blackened circles are carriers with such linkage (primary active transport pumps). Gaps in cell membranes represent ion channels. c.a., carbonic anhydrase. The arrow between cells indicates the paracellular shunt pathway. Note that the potassium ions taken up by the basolateral sodium–potassium pump 'recycle' across that membrane via a potassium channel.

is the Na,K-dependent ATPase located along the basolateral (blood-facing) membrane of the proximal tubular cells. This pump lowers the sodium concentration inside the cell to around 5–10 mmol/L, thereby creating a marked electrochemical gradient for the entry of sodium from the tubular fluid (where it is present in plasma-like concentrations) across the apical cell membrane into the cell. Located in this membrane are several carrier proteins through which sodium entry is coupled with the transport of other solutes, which themselves move against their electrochemical gradient (or 'uphill') by what is termed secondary active transport.

Two types of such carriers are particularly important. One group mediates the cotransport of a variety of organic solutes from the luminal fluid in conjunction with sodium. In this group are a number of carrier molecules, each with specificity for a different substance, e.g. a sodium–glucose cotransporter, a family of related sodium–amino acid cotransporters, a sodium–phosphate cotransporter, and so on.

A second carrier type mediates the countertransport of an absorbed sodium ion with a hydrogen ion produced within the epithelial cell. This sodium–hydrogen exchanger (NHE-3) is one of a family of such proteins having widespread ramifications for cellular acid–base metabolism, and is important in the mechanism of proximal bicarbonate reabsorption (see Chapter 4).

While these and other mechanisms for the movement of sodium into the proximal tubular cells from the luminal fluid are well documented, they can account for only a fraction of the total reabsorptive flux of sodium which occurs across the epithelium. More than half of this sodium movement appears to occur between adjacent epithelial cells, through what is termed the 'shunt' pathway. A component of this flux is driven by transepithelial electrical gradients, but some sodium and other ions are carried across the tubular wall by 'solvent drag', pulled in the bulk flow of water which is known to occur through the intercellular pathway. This water flux itself is driven partly by the small but significant osmotic (and oncotic) gradients established across the proximal tubular wall along its length, and partly by a small hydrostatic pressure gradient favouring fluid movement from the tubular lumen into the peritubular capillaries.

Loop of Henle

The cells of the thin descending limb of the loop of Henle do not carry out active transepithelial ion transport, but act as important passive equilibrators in the process of countercurrent multiplication (see Chapter 3). The thick ascending limb segment, on the other hand, is responsible for reabsorption of a further 25% of the filtered load of sodium, and contributes importantly to the build-up of the medullary interstitial concentration gradient which is essential in the mechanism for ultimate concentration of the urine (see Chapter 3).

The transport properties of the thick ascending limb include the following:

- Extensive transepithelial reabsorption of sodium and chloride is accompanied by smaller fluxes of potassium, magnesium and calcium.

- This nephron segment is impermeable to water under all conditions.

- Transport of all ions across this segment is powerfully inhibited by loop-acting diuretic drugs such as furosemide (frusemide).

- A small lumen-positive transepithelial potential difference normally exists across this segment.

Studies of the mechanism of ion transport in the thick ascending limb have given rise to the cell model shown in Fig. 2.7. As in the proximal tubule, the primary active transport step is the Na,K-ATPase located on the basolateral cell membrane. In this cell, however, sodium entry from the luminal fluid across the apical cell membrane is via a quite different mechanism than that operating in the proximal tubule. Here, one sodium ion, one potassium ion and two chloride ions interact with a carrier protein molecule embedded in the apical cell membrane ('the triple cotransporter', or NKCCT). It is this carrier whose function is blocked by loop diuretics such as furosemide (frusemide), which therefore results in the inhibition of the reabsorptive activity of this segment. Note that the movement of sodium into the cell via this carrier is electrochemically 'downhill', but is coupled through the action of the carrier to the uphill transport of chloride and potassium. Of the potassium accumulated inside the cell, some is transported out of the cell across the basolateral membrane, in part coupled with chloride, resulting in net reabsorption of potassium across the epithelium. However, a component of intracellular potassium recycles

Fig. 2.7 Principal transport properties of a cell in the thick ascending limb of the loop of Henle. The ⊕ indicates that the transepithelial electrical potential difference is positive in the lumen relative to the blood side. The carrier marked F ⤵ is the molecular target of the diuretic furosemide and related drugs. Symbol conventions as in Fig. 2.6. See text for detailed description.

Fig. 2.8 Principal transport properties of an early distal tubule (distal convoluted tubule) cell. The lumen is electrically positive with respect to the blood side. The carrier marked T ⤵ is the molecular target of thiazides and related diuretic drugs. Symbol conventions as in Fig. 2.6. See text for detailed description.

through a potassium channel in the apical cell membrane into the lumen, where it becomes available for re-entry into the cell through the triple cotransporter. It should be noted that there is considerable flux of cations such as sodium, potassium, calcium and magnesium across this epithelium via the shunt pathway between adjacent cells, driven largely by the lumen-positive transepithelial potential difference.

The fact that this tubular segment is impermeable to water under all conditions means that it acts as a site of dilution of the luminal fluid, i.e. removal of electrolytes but not water lowers the luminal osmolality. At the same time, however, the segment plays a vital role in building the concentrating capacity of the renal medulla, as will be explained in the next chapter. It is therefore a critical portion of the nephron not only for net electrolyte re-absorption, but in contributing to the regulation of the osmolality of the body fluids. All of these processes are disrupted by agents such as loop diuretics which interfere with the operation of this segment.

Distal tubule

The transport properties of the early distal tubule (or distal convoluted tubule) include the following:

- Sodium is reabsorbed with chloride but with little net potassium movement.
- Water permeability is very low under all conditions.
- A further component of filtered calcium is reabsorbed.
- Sodium transport is inhibited by thiazides and related drugs.

The cell model which has been developed to explain the operation of this segment is shown in Fig. 2.8. Again, the primary active transport step is the operation of the

Na,K-ATPase in the basolateral membrane. There is again a passive gradient for sodium to enter the cell from the luminal fluid across the apical cell membrane, and in this segment this uptake step is mediated by a sodium–chloride cotransport carrier molecule (called the NCT), in which one sodium and one chloride ion are taken up simultaneously. It is this carrier whose function is blocked by the thiazide diuretics and related molecules, resulting in the loss of unreabsorbed sodium chloride into the urine.

While no significant potassium fluxes occur across this cell segment, transepithelial calcium reabsorption does occur by the mechanisms shown in Fig. 2.8. This involves uptake of calcium across the apical cell membrane via a calcium channel, with extrusion of calcium across the basolateral membrane via a sodium–calcium counter-transport carrier, driven by the passive inward movement of sodium from the ECF. Thus, during thiazide action, sodium entry into the cell is inhibited, resulting in a lowering of intracellular sodium by the continued action of the basolateral Na,K-ATPase. This in turn increases the activity of the basal sodium–calcium exchanger, resulting in lower cell calcium and thus enhanced entry of calcium through the apical membrane, and hence across the epithelium. This may explain the apparent paradox of treatment with thiazide diuretics during which sodium excretion is increased but calcium excretion is decreased, although other mechanisms (such as enhanced calcium reabsorption with sodium in the proximal tubule secondary to mild hypovolaemia after thiazide action) may also be involved.

Cortical collecting duct

The late segment of the distal tubule has similar transport properties to the earliest part of the collecting duct system, formed where two distal tubular segments join together. These properties continue until the collecting duct leaves the cortex to become the medullary collecting duct.

The transport properties of this nephron segment include the following:

- There is reabsorption of some 2–3% of the filtered sodium load, accompanied in part by chloride reabsorption, potassium secretion and acid secretion into the lumen.

- All of these transport processes are stimulated by the circulating steroid hormone aldosterone.

- Water permeability of this segment is variable, being increased by circulating antidiuretic hormone (vasopressin).

- Sodium reabsorption in this segment is inhibited by amiloride and (when aldosterone is acting) spironolactone; when these drugs are present, secretion of both K^+ and H^+ is reduced.

- There is normally an appreciable lumen-negative transepithelial potential difference, but this is largely abolished by the action of amiloride and spironolactone.

The cell mechanisms which have been proposed to account for these transport properties are shown in Fig. 2.9. There are two distinct cell types defined histologically in this segment, mediating different transport functions.

The principal cells are the site of sodium reabsorption and potassium secretion. Again the primary active transport step driving these processes is the basolateral Na,K-ATPase. Sodium enters the cell from the luminal fluid down its electrochemical gradient, passing in this instance through a channel called the epithelial sodium channel, or ENaC. This step generates a lumen-negative

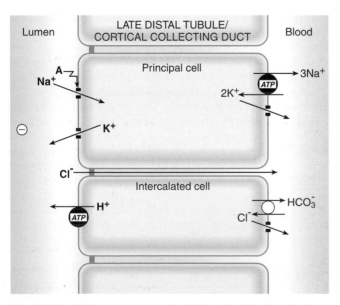

Fig. 2.9 Principal transport properties of the cells of the late distal tubule/cortical collecting duct. The lumen is electrically negative with respect to the blood side. The channel marked A ⌐ᵧ is the site of action of the diuretic amiloride. Symbol conventions as in Fig. 2.6. See text for detailed description.

diffusion potential. Potassium accumulated in the cell moves into the luminal fluid through an apical potassium channel, down its electrochemical gradient. This cell type is also known to be a target for the action of aldosterone, which enters the cell from the blood, and interacts with a receptor molecule located in the cytoplasm. The hormone–receptor complex undergoes translocation into the nucleus, after which transcription and translation of aldosterone-induced proteins occurs, resulting in activation of all the transport steps undertaken by this cell. In addition, this cell contains basolateral membrane receptors for circulating vasopressin, the action of which results in increased transepithelial water transport in this segment (see also Chapter 3).

The intercalated cells are the site of acid secretion into the lumen within this tubular segment. This is mediated by an active hydrogen pump, the H^+-ATPase, located on the apical cell membrane, which translocates hydrogen ions from the cell cytoplasm into the lumen. These hydrogen ions are generated within the cell by the action of carbonic anhydrase, which catalyses the formation of carbonic acid from water and carbon dioxide. This disassociates into a hydrogen ion which is secreted into the lumen and a bicarbonate ion which enters the ECF across the basolateral membrane, in exchange for chloride via an anion countertransporter ('anion exchanger 1'). This process of acid secretion is also activated by aldosterone.

This nephron segment is sensitive to a number of transport inhibitors. Amiloride blocks the apical sodium channel in the principal cells. This results not only in inhibition of sodium reabsorption, but also greatly reduces potassium and acid secretion, which are partly dependent on the negative lumen potential generated by sodium reabsorption. Spironolactone blocks the binding of aldosterone to its cytoplasmic receptor, thereby interfering with the activation by aldosterone of sodium reabsorption, potassium secretion and acid secretion.

It should be mentioned that, under unusual metabolic conditions, namely potassium depletion and alkalosis, this nephron segment is able to adapt its transport functions to mediate potassium reabsorption and bicarbonate secretion (respectively), though these processes are not active under normal dietary and metabolic conditions.

Regulation of sodium transport

A number of mechanisms interact to ensure that sodium excretion by the kidney is appropriately matched to changes in sodium intake and the ECF volume. These mechanisms require the precisely balanced operation of various sensory systems which detect changes in the ECF volume (and related parameters), and a number of effector mechanisms capable of altering the kidney's sodium excretion rate.

The sensing mechanisms include:

- Volume receptors in the cardiac atria and intrathoracic veins.

- Pressure receptors in the central arterial tree and the afferent arterioles within the kidney.

- Tubular fluid NaCl concentration receptors within the distal nephron (the macula densa).

The intrathoracic volume receptors respond to reduced distension by signalling to the brainstem that central venous volume has fallen, resulting in activation of effector mechanisms to restore the volume and pressure within the circulation. The opposite responses take place during ECF volume expansion. In addition, during volume expansion increased stretch of the cardiac atria directly results in the release of atrial natriuretic peptide (see below). Other afferents arise from arterial basoreceptors in the aortic arch and carotid sinus and these give signals paralleling those of the volume receptors in most circumstances. The operation of the intrarenal baroreceptors and the macula densa is explained below in the section on the renin–angiotensin–aldosterone system.

The effector mechanisms involved in adjusting renal sodium excretion are summarized in Table 2.3.

Of the neurohumoral mechanisms, the most important is the renin–angiotensin–aldosterone (RAA) system. As illustrated in Fig. 2.10, this system is activated by stimuli leading to the release of renin, an enzyme contained within specialized smooth muscle cells in the walls of the afferent and efferent arterioles. The principal stimuli to its release are as follows:

- Reduced perfusion pressure in the afferent arteriole.

- Increased sympathetic nerve activity in fibres innervating the afferent and efferent arterioles.

- Decreased sodium chloride concentration flowing through the distal tubule.

The inset in Fig. 2.10 shows the anatomical arrangements whereby the afferent and efferent arterioles of a given nephron come into direct contact with the earliest part of that nephron's distal tubule, where the epithelial cells become modified to form the macula densa. This juxtaglomerular apparatus brings together the three principal stimuli promoting renin release: thus when ECF volume is low, the pressure distending the afferent arteriole falls, sympathetic nerve discharges to the renin-containing cells increase, and sodium concentration in the distal tubular lumen falls because of activated sodium reabsorption in earlier tubular segments.

The renin released into the circulation acts to cleave the peptide substrate angiotensinogen (manufactured in the liver), producing angiotensin I in the circulation. After passage through capillary beds, notably in the lungs, this is cleaved by angiotensin-converting enzyme into angiotensin II. This octapeptide is the central mediator of the RAA system, having multiple actions:

- It directly acts to vasoconstrict small arterioles.

- It directly stimulates proximal tubular sodium reabsorption.

- It causes the zona glomerulosa cells of the adrenal cortex to release the steroid hormone aldosterone.

As described earlier in this chapter, aldosterone acts to stimulate salt reabsorption in the cortical collecting duct

Table 2.3 Effector mechanisms involved in regulation of renal sodium transport

Effector system	Site of action	Net effect of activation
Neurohumoral mechanisms		
Renin–angiotensin–aldosterone system	PT (angiotensin II), causing increased Na reabsorption CCD (aldosterone), causing increased Na reabsorption	Decreased Na excretion
Sympathetic nervous system/catecholamines	PT (noradrenaline; norepinephrine), causing increased Na reabsorption	Decreased Na excretion
Atrial natriuretic peptide	Glomerulus, causing increased GFR PT, causing decreased Na reabsorption MCD, causing decreased Na reabsorption	Increased Na excretion
Natriuretic hormone	PT, causing decreased Na reabsorption	Increased Na excretion
Prostaglandins	Glomerulus, causing increased GFR TAL and CCD, causing decreased Na reabsorption	Increased Na excretion
Haemodynamic-mechanical mechanisms		
GFR changes	Glomerulus	Increased GFR causes increased Na excretion
Peritubular physical forces (hydrostatic and oncotic pressures in the peritubular capillaries)	PT	Increased filtration fraction causes decreased Na excretion

Note that the table excludes a number of mediators of altered sodium transport whose physiological role is not well established. PT, proximal tubule; CCD, cortical collecting duct (including late distal tubules forming initial collecting duct); TAL, thick ascending limb of the loop of Henle; MCD, medullary collecting duct; GFR, glomerular filtration rate.

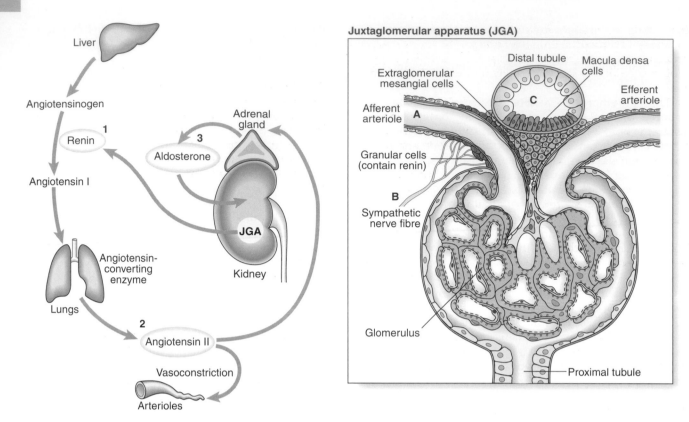

Fig. 2.10 The renin–angiotensin–aldosterone system. The numbers 1–3 show the sequence of steps in the activation of the system. The inset shows the juxtaglomerular apparatus (JGA) with the three major stimuli acting as triggers for renin release: A, fall in pressure in afferent arteriole; B, release of noradrenaline (norepinephrine) by sympathetic nerve endings on granular cells; C, fall in NaCl concentration in distal tubule. Note that angiotensin II has a number of additional actions not shown on this figure (see text).

of the nephron, hence reducing sodium and water excretion from the kidney. The net effect of these actions is to restore blood pressure and ECF volume towards normal, thereby decreasing the stimulus which led to the activation of the system.

The sympathetic nervous system is also involved in the response to hypovolaemia, not only by acting as a stimulus for renin release, described above, but also by releasing noradrenaline (norepinephrine) around the proximal tubular cells, where it directly stimulates tubular sodium reabsorption. In addition, sympathetic activation vasoconstricts the afferent arteriole, reducing GFR and further limiting sodium and fluid losses.

Most of the other humoral mechanisms involved in sodium regulation lead to an increase in sodium excretion, thereby playing an important role in defending against volume expansion during periods of high salt availability.

Atrial natriuretic peptide is released from the cardiac atria when they undergo stretch during high volume states. It circulates as a peptide containing 28 amino acids and has numerous actions contributing to enhanced sodium excretion:

- The GFR is increased, via an action of atrial natriuretic peptide to dilate the afferent arterioles.

- Sodium reabsorption by the proximal tubule and medullary collecting duct is inhibited.

- Secretion of renin and aldosterone is reduced, further switching off sodium-retaining systems.

A less well defined mediator of sodium excretion during volume expansion is the natriuretic hormone released from the brain during these conditions. It is known to have ouabain- or digoxin-like properties in that it inhibits Na,K-ATPase in both vascular smooth muscle and renal epithelial cells. In the former, the result is an increase in intracellular sodium and calcium concentrations leading to vasoconstriction, while in the kidney the effect is an inhibition of sodium reabsorption, promoting natriuresis (increased sodium excretion).

A variety of other intrarenal mediators are involved in inhibiting sodium reabsorption under certain physiological conditions, and of these the most important clinically is the intrarenal prostaglandin (PG) system. Locally acting prostaglandins, PGE_2 in particular, are known to enhance glomerular filtration and decrease sodium reabsorption in the thick ascending limb of the loop of Henle and in the cortical collecting duct, the net effect being enhancement of sodium excretion. Other systems which have been implicated in sodium transport regulation include dopamine, kinins, adenosine/ATP, nitric oxide and endothelin. The role of these mediators under physiological conditions is incompletely defined at the present time.

Another important system involved in the response to major (5–10%) changes in circulating volume is antidiuretic hormone. This effector peptide acts both to increase water reabsorption from the nephron and to vasoconstrict blood vessels, with little direct effect on sodium balance. It will be described in more detail in Chapter 3.

Haemodynamic and mechanical mechanisms are also involved in the maintenance of sodium balance. Changes in GFR are involved in mediating the actions of some of the neurohumoral mechanisms outlined above. Minor minute-to-minute changes in GFR are usually not a determinant of sodium excretion, largely because of the phenomenon of glomerulotubular balance: this describes the proportional adjustment of proximal reabsorption to shifts in GFR, minimizing the net excretory effect of such changes. During wider swings in circulating blood volume, proximal tubular reabsorption is thought to be altered by changes in the physical forces affecting sodium and fluid reabsorption from the proximal tubule, namely the hydrostatic and oncotic pressures in the peritubular capillaries. See 2.1: 3.

Looking first at Joanne's urea, creatinine and urate results, we note that the urea and urate are elevated, while the creatinine is within the normal range. As will be discussed further in Chapter 5, creatinine acts as a marker of the GFR, and the fact that it is not significantly elevated suggests that the GFR has not fallen greatly (though a small rise in creatinine within the normal range cannot be excluded). The increase in plasma urea is consistent with hypovolaemia, since urea is handled by the kidney both by filtration and by partial reabsorption within the nephron, the extent of which is increased during low volume states (a number of other factors can influence the plasma urea, as described in Chapter 5).

The increase in plasma urate (the anion base of uric acid) is also suggestive of volume depletion. This nitrogenous breakdown product of nucleic acid metabolism is freely filtered at the glomerulus, but undergoes both extensive reabsorption from and secretion into the proximal tubule, usually resulting in a final excretion of some 10% of the filtered urate load. However, during volume contraction, the forces promoting increased proximal tubular sodium and fluid reabsorption also increase the absorptive component of proximal urate transport, resulting in elevated plasma urate concentration. Indeed, in susceptible individuals, this can result in an attack of gout because of uric acid crystallization in joint tissues and the resulting inflammation.

Joanne's electrolyte results show that the sodium and chloride concentrations are normal, while the potassium concentration is reduced and the bicarbonate concentration elevated. It is important to recognize that the normal sodium concentration does not reflect a normal total body sodium, as indeed we have concluded that she has

---

Body fluids and nephron function: 3

Biochemistry results

We can now understand that Joanne's symptoms and signs of volume depletion have resulted from the action of the furosemide (frusemide) tablets she had been taking, resulting in inhibition of sodium reabsorption in the loop of Henle, and hence negative net sodium balance.

Further investigation included the following biochemistry results:

Sodium 136 mmol/L
*Potassium 2.7 mmol/L
Chloride 95 mmol/L
*Bicarbonate 32 mmol/L
*Urea 10.5 mmol/L
Creatinine 0.12 mmol/L
*Urate 0.48 mmol/L.

These results lead us to the following question:
How have the abnormalities in her biochemical profile come about?

*Results outside the normal range; see Appendix.

---

been partly depleted of sodium because of the action of the diuretic. The normal concentration simply reflects the fact that water loss from the ECF has been roughly proportionate to sodium, resulting in no net change in the ECF sodium concentration or osmolality. (Disturbances of sodium concentration may be seen during diuretic treatment under certain conditions, as discussed in the next chapter.)

To understand the origin of the hypokalaemia, we need to review mechanisms regulating potassium balance.

Potassium transport

Potassium is freely filtered at the glomerulus and, like sodium, some 65% of the filtered amount is reabsorbed in the proximal tubule. Again paralleling sodium, about 25% more is reabsorbed in the thick ascending limb of the loop of Henle. While no potassium is transported in the early (convoluted) distal tubule, in the late distal tubule joining the cortical collecting duct potassium is actually transported into the tubular fluid by a process of secretion. This secretory step is carried out by the mechanisms illustrated in Fig. 2.9 – the principal cell of the cortical collecting duct.

Under conditions of low potassium intake, the extent of secretion may be minimal, resulting in a net fractional excretion of potassium of some 10% of the filtered load. During potassium depletion, net reabsorption from the cortical and medullary collecting duct can even occur, resulting in fractional excretion rates as low as 5%. More commonly, however, under normal dietary conditions or during potassium loading, potassium secretion can be stimulated such that the final urine contains 20% or more of the filtered potassium amount.

The factors regulating the extent of potassium secretion in the cortical collecting duct segment include:

- Circulating factors
  - high plasma aldosterone concentration
  - high plasma potassium concentration
  - high plasma pH.

- Luminal factors
  - high sodium delivery rate
  - high luminal flow rate
  - negative lumen potential difference.

Aldosterone acts as the key regulator of potassium balance, in parallel with its role in sodium metabolism but mediated by a quite different feedback mechanism. As shown in Fig. 2.11, a high plasma potassium concentration resulting from increased dietary potassium or other reasons directly stimulates the zona glomerulosa cells of the adrenal cortex to secrete aldosterone, which, by increasing potassium secretion into the distal nephron, leads to increased potassium excretion, thereby reducing the high plasma potassium. This is the main negative feedback mechanism responsible for maintaining the plasma potassium within the range 3.5–5.0 mmol/L.

Of the luminal factors, the rate of delivery of sodium and fluid from the earlier nephron segments is an important determinant of potassium secretion because of their influence on the transport processes of the cortical collecting duct.

From the above, it can be seen why a diuretic drug acting to inhibit loop of Henle sodium reabsorption would lead to potassium depletion. The following factors may be involved:

- The potassium normally reabsorbed across the thick ascending limb is lost into the urine.

- The sodium not reabsorbed in the loop passes through to the distal tubule and cortical collecting duct where it is available for increased exchange for potassium through the principal cell mechanisms.

- The increased flow of fluid accompanying sodium through the distal potassium-secretory segment dilutes the luminal fluid and so provides an increased gradient for potassium to move into the lumen.

- The volume depletion resulting from diuretic action stimulates aldosterone (via renin and angiotensin), further amplifying potassium secretion.

Hypokalaemia can be caused by a variety of other disturbances, as shown in Box 2.2. Note that in some cases the low ECF potassium concentration results largely from a shift into the larger ICF pool. When external losses do occur, this may be from either the gastrointestinal tract or the kidney. Frequently, losses occur from both systems since, when there is a reduction in ECF volume, aldosterone promotes potassium secretion in the kidney and hence increases urinary potassium excretion.

The increase in plasma bicarbonate in Joanne's case reflects a mild metabolic alkalosis, largely owing to the enhancement of hydrogen ion secretion resulting from increased sodium delivery through the cortical collecting duct segment, as outlined above. Again, enhancement of this step by high levels of aldosterone serves to aggravate this loss of acid.

Box 2.2 Causes of hypokalaemia

- **Redistribution into cells**
  e.g. alkalosis, catecholamines, insulin excess, hypokalaemic periodic paralysis
- **Inadequate K intake**
  e.g. starvation, inadequate replacement after operation
- **Increased external K losses**
  Gastrointestinal tract:
  e.g. vomiting, diarrhoea, laxative abuse, villous adenoma of rectum
  Kidney:
  e.g. high mineralocorticoid activity (hyperaldosteronism, steroid therapy, etc.), diuretics, classic (distal) renal tubular acidosis, congenital tubular transport disorders (Bartter's and Gitelman's syndromes)

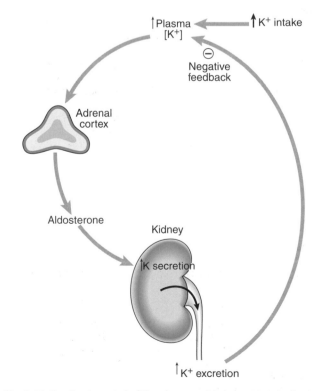

Fig. 2.11 Feedback control of the plasma potassium concentration.

Pharmacology of diuretic agents

This chapter has introduced the mechanisms of action of a number of commonly used diuretic drugs. For completion, a summary of the major agents in clinical use, together with their principal properties and actions, is given in Tables 2.4 and 2.5.

An important generalization about most of the drugs used as diuretics is that they act on the mechanism for sodium uptake from the luminal fluid across the apical cell membrane in a particular tubular segment. This gives rise to the specificity of their site of action, given that the apical uptake step is mediated by different mechanisms in each segment, as described earlier. In contrast, the sodium exit step from the base of the cells is the same in each tubular segment, namely the Na,K-ATPase pump.

One group of diuretic drugs not shown in the accompanying tables is the osmotic diuretics. These substances are freely filtered but are not reabsorbed by any part of the tubular system. Their action is thus not site-specific in that they entrain fluid osmotically within the tubular lumen and therefore limit the extent of sodium reabsorption in multiple segments. The principal clinical example of such an agent is mannitol, which must be given by intravenous infusion, and is used to achieve short-term diuresis in conditions associated with cell swelling, such as cerebral oedema.

All the other diuretic drugs detailed in the tables (except spironolactone) must be delivered into the luminal fluid in appreciable concentrations to affect the apical sodium transport mechanisms. Delivery to the site of action is achieved partly by filtration, but there is an important component of active secretion of the diuretic molecules across the proximal tubular epithelium, mediated by the transport mechanisms available to secrete weak organic acids and bases in this nephron segment. This is of particular importance in determining the pharmacokinetics of these drugs since most are strongly protein-bound in the plasma, a property which itself leads to a very low delivery rate into the tubule by glomerular filtration alone.

More background information concerning the action of carbonic anhydrase inhibitors and the effects of diuretics on concentrating and diluting capacity is given in the subsequent two chapters of this volume.

Interesting facts

An extract from the foxglove plant, now known to contain digitalis, a cardiac glycoside related to digoxin, was used in the 18th and 19th centuries as a treatment for oedema (then called dropsy) in the belief that it acted on the kidney as a diuretic agent. It is now known that the diuretic action results instead from an improvement in the force of cardiac contraction caused by the drug, with a consequent increase in cardiac output, renal perfusion and hence GFR.

Table 2.4 Summary of sites and mechanisms of action of the principal classes of diuretic drugs

Site	Drug class	Prototype drug	Mechanism of action
Proximal tubule	Carbonic anhydrase inhibitors	Acetazolamide	Prevent $NaHCO_3$ reabsorption by limiting H formation
Thick ascending limb of loop of Henle	'Loop' diuretics	Furosemide (frusemide)	Block apical Na, K, 2Cl cotransporter
Early distal tubule	Thiazides and related drugs	Chlorothiazide	Block apical Na, Cl cotransporter
Late distal tubule/cortical collecting duct	a. Sodium channel blockers b. Aldosterone antagonists	a. Amiloride b. Spironolactone	a. Block apical Na channel b. Block aldosterone receptor in cytoplasm

Table 2.5 Effects of diuretics on renal electrolyte and water excretion

Diuretic class	Na excretion*	K excretion	Anion excreted	Concentrating capacity†	Diluting capacity†
Carbonic anhydrase inhibitors	5	Increased	HCO_3^-	Increased	Increased
Loop blockers	20	Increased	Cl^-	Decreased	Decreased
Thiazides	6	Increased	Cl^-	No change	Decreased
K-sparing drugs	2	Decreased	Cl^-/HCO_3^-	No change	No change

*Maximum percentage of filtered load of Na excreted into the urine during diuretic action.

†Effect of the diuretic on the capacity of the kidney to concentrate and dilute the urine (see Chapter 3).

Clinical use of diuretics

The two commonest indications for diuretic prescription are in the treatment of hypertension (see Chapter 9) and in the reduction of ECF volume in oedematous states (see Chapter 6).

Diuretic use is frequently complicated by a number of adverse effects, which are summarized in Box 2.3. These fall broadly into three categories: physiologically predictable side effects (including abnormal plasma electrolyte concentrations), metabolic side effects (including effects on glucose and lipid metabolism, where the mechanism is poorly defined), and allergic or idiosyncratic reactions. The latter are most prominent with drugs in the sulphonamide class, including carbonic anhydrase inhibitors, furosemide (frusemide) and the thiazides.

There are a number of indications for the rational prescription of combinations of diuretic drugs. First, to reduce an unwanted electrolyte effect such as hypokalaemia induced by one class of agents (loop and early distal drugs), simultaneous treatment with a potassium-sparing drug such as amiloride can lead to a more neutral net effect on potassium balance while maintaining adequate diuretic action. Second, in resistant oedema associated with advanced disease of the heart or kidneys, it is sometimes appropriate to coadminister drugs acting at multiple sites along the nephron to counter the 'resistance' which may develop to one agent because of compensatory enhancement of sodium reabsorption by more

Box 2.3 Adverse effects of diuretic drug use

'Physiological' side effects

Hypovolaemia
Hyponatraemia
Hypokalaemia*
Metabolic alkalosis*
Hyperuricaemia
Hypomagnesaemia*
Hypocalcaemia (loop-acting drugs only)

Metabolic side effects

Glucose intolerance/hyperglycaemia
Hyperlipidaemia

Miscellaneous side effects

Hypersensitivity reactions
Acute pancreatitis/cholecystitis (thiazides)
Impotence

The effects shown apply chiefly to the loop and early distal acting drugs.

*These effects are not seen with drugs acting in the cortical collecting duct; these may cause the opposite side effects (hyperkalaemia and metabolic acidosis). Carbonic anhydrase inhibitors may cause hypokalaemia with metabolic acidosis.

---

distally located segments. In these circumstances the prescriber must take particular care to avoid complications resulting from uncontrolled losses of fluid and electrolytes by careful clinical and laboratory monitoring.

In general, the following summarizes the guidelines for diuretic use under most conditions:

- Use the minimum effective dose.
- Use for as short a period of time as necessary.
- Monitor regularly for adverse effects.
- Use only for appropriate indications.

With regard to the last point, Joanne's use of diuretics for cosmetic or weight control purposes is clearly inappropriate.

Principles of fluid and electrolyte replacement therapy

The key steps in correcting a disturbance in body fluid and electrolyte composition are:

1. Cessation or reversal of the causative disturbance.
2. Replacement of estimated deficits.
3. Provision of ongoing maintenance requirements.

Where the dominant clinical problem relates to an inadequate circulating blood volume, the chief goal is to restore the circulation by supplying fluid that will be held preferentially in the circulating compartment of the ECF, that is, the plasma.

Three basic types of replacement fluid are available for clinical use:

- Electrolyte-free sugar solutions (e.g. 5% D-glucose in water).
- Isotonic solutions of sodium salts (e.g. 0.9% sodium chloride, which is 150 mM NaCl or normal saline).
- Isotonic salt solutions containing colloid macromolecules (e.g. semi-synthetic gelatins).

The effectiveness of each of these solutions in restoring circulating volume can be deduced by reference to Fig. 2.3. Using first principles, considering 1 litre of each solution infused into a vein, the approximate distribution of volume would be as follows:

- The 5% dextrose solution would distribute approximately as does total body water, given that glucose is taken up freely by most cellular tissues. This would result in minimal expansion of the circulating blood volume, since the entire plasma and red cell volume is only about 12.5% of the total body water.
- A litre of normal saline would remain largely confined to the ECF, but of this only some 20% would remain in the plasma, the rest moving into the interstitial fluid compartment.

- A litre of colloid-containing solution would be largely retained in the plasma compartment, since the oncotic effect of the colloid macromolecule would serve to hold the added fluid inside the capillary endothelial barrier.

The urgency of fluid replacement and the choice of fluid used depends very much on the clinical circumstances, including the rate of development and nature of the deficit, assessed by clinical and biochemical parameters. Many cases of mild or chronic fluid and electrolyte deficiency can be corrected by simple measures, involving cessation of the causative disturbance, and oral replacement of fluid and electrolytes found to be deficient. In more acute or severe situations, intravenous therapy will be necessary. In either case, attention needs also to be given to prevent recurrence of the initiating disturbance.

Case 2.1 Body fluids and nephron function: 4

Treatment

The clinicians caring for Joanne considered that her circulation was significantly affected by her prolonged diuretic use, and that a period of intravenous therapy would be the most effective way of restoring her circulation. She was admitted to hospital and the diuretics were ceased. She was given 1 litre of normal saline intravenously every 12 h for 48 h, with 30 mmol potassium chloride added to each litre.

Her symptoms rapidly resolved, and her plasma biochemistry normalized. She received counselling about the importance of refraining from further use of diuretic medications, and was given support and advice about her perceived weight and swelling problems. Her family doctor was involved in following her up in these matters.

WATER BALANCE AND REGULATION OF OSMOLALITY

3

Chapter objectives

After studying this chapter you should be able to:

1. Define the normal range for plasma osmolality.

2. Outline the mechanisms by which the kidney can concentrate the urine (during underhydration) and dilute the urine (during overhydration).

3. Explain the feedback mechanisms for the control of plasma osmolality, and the role of vasopressin (antidiuretic hormone).

4. Outline the differential diagnosis of polyuria, and explain some mechanisms involved in conditions associated with impaired capacity to concentrate the urine.

5. Give a differential diagnosis of hypernatraemia.

6. Describe the mechanisms involved in conditions involving impaired ability to dilute the urine.

7. Give a differential diagnosis of hyponatraemia.

Introduction

The previous chapter was largely concerned with the mechanisms whereby the kidney regulates body sodium balance. The point was made that the volume of the extracellular fluid (ECF) is largely determined by body sodium content, and hence adjustments to the renal sodium excretion rate have a major bearing on the ECF volume. We explained that, for the most part, alterations in tubular sodium transport are accompanied by parallel movements of water (though not necessarily in the same tubular segment) such that no net change in body fluid osmolality generally results from these adjustments.

In this chapter, we consider the mechanisms whereby water is handled by the kidney, independent of movements of sodium. These principles will give rise to an understanding of how the kidney is able to concentrate the urine by retaining water, or dilute the urine by excreting water as circumstances demand. It will also lead to an understanding of the origin of the clinical problems of polyuria, hypernatraemia and hyponatraemia. See 3.1:1.

Causes and assessment of polyuria

In principle, a high urine flow rate may be produced either by a primary increase in solute excretion or by a primary increase in water excretion.

Polyuria caused by solute diuresis results from the delivery of a high load of solute through the nephron, either as a result of filtration of a poorly reabsorbed solute, or of blunted reabsorption of a solute normally transported out of the tubular fluid. (Note that increased glomerular filtration rate (GFR) *per se* is not a common cause of polyuria, largely because of glomerulotubular balance; see Chapter 2). The first mechanism applies to the osmotic diuresis produced by infusions of mannitol, which cannot be reabsorbed from the nephron and hence traps water osmotically within the tubular lumen, resulting in a high urine flow rate. Osmotic diuresis can also occur during disease states, notably in uncontrolled diabetes mellitus. In this case, increased plasma glucose concentrations result in the filtration of a glucose load greater than that which can be reabsorbed by the proximal tubule glucose reabsorption mechanism (saturation of the sodium–glucose cotransport carrier), leading to **glycosuria** accompanied by increased water flow because of the osmotic effect of the glucose trapped in the lumen. This mechanism accounts for the polyuria and dehydration encountered in newly presenting or uncontrolled insulin-dependent diabetes. A broadly similar mechanism is occasionally seen during the development of chronic kidney disease, where high levels of urea have a diuretic effect.

The second mechanism for solute diuresis is that produced by the commonly used diuretic drugs, which act to block the specific mechanisms for sodium reabsorption in discrete segments of the nephron (see Chapter 2).

A case of polyuria

Robert Underwood is a 46-year-old man who presents to a doctor in a suburban medical centre complaining of passing large volumes of urine which is virtually colourless ('like water'), accompanied by excessive thirst. He claims to be drinking 5 or more litres of water per day, and passing similar volumes of urine. These symptoms have been troubling him for several weeks. He denies a history of similar complaints in the past, and has never been diagnosed with diabetes. He has never had known kidney disease and states that his general health has been good, although he has had some 'emotional problems' over the years. The family history is unremarkable. He says he is a reformed smoker, and does not drink alcohol at all.

On examination he seems a little agitated but otherwise looks quite well. The skin, lips and mouth appear rather dry, but the blood pressure is normal at 130/80, the pulse 84 beats/min. The rest of the examination is normal. A urine specimen is obtained, which is a very pale colour, and on urinalysis proves to be negative for glucose, blood and protein. This specimen, as well as a sample of blood, is sent to the pathology laboratory.

The questions that arise in considering this case are:

1. What might be causing his polyuria and thirst?
2. What determines how concentrated the urine is under normal conditions?

Polyuria of this cause is most prominent soon after commencement of the diuretic drug.

Water-based or dilute polyuria has a quite different mechanism, and can arise in one of two ways. First, a high intake of water will lead directly to a high output of dilute urine, through mechanisms to be described in this chapter. While a history of excessive water drinking might be expected in this situation, covert overdrinking is sometimes encountered in patients with psychiatric disturbances (psychogenic polydipsia). An alternative mechanism for polyuria associated with dilute urine is when the primary disorder involves the kidney's inability to concentrate the urine normally. The physiological defects giving rise to this condition, known as diabetes insipidus, will be detailed further below.

Table 3.1 illustrates some differential features in the diagnostic approach to polyuria. Of particular interest in this case and for the subject matter of this chapter, is the differentiation between the two forms of water diuresis. While in both forms the urine is dilute with low osmolality, in the case where the diuresis is being driven by high water intake the plasma would be expected to have a low osmolality, resulting directly from excessive water reabsorption from the gut. In the case of impaired urinary concentration

Table 3.1 Diagnostic approach to polyuria

Type	Examples	Plasma	Urine
Solute	Uncontrolled diabetes mellitus (solute = glucose)	Increased osmolality, hyperglycaemia	High osmolality, glycosuria
	Furosemide (frusemide) therapy (solute = NaCl)	Normal osmolality*	Variable osmolality, high Na
Water	Psychogenic polydipsia	Low–normal osmolality	Low osmolality
	Impaired urine concentration (central or nephrogenic DI)	High–normal osmolality	Low osmolality

*The plasma osmolality and sodium concentration may be normal, low or high during loop diuretic therapy, depending on the water intake. DI, diabetes insipidus.

mechanisms, the plasma osmolality would be high since the primary problem is excessive loss of water from the ECF into the urine.

By reference to Table 3.1, Mr Underwood's polyuria cannot be attributed to glucose or sodium as solutes, but is a water diuresis. Since the plasma sodium and osmolality are above the normal range, we can deduce that his problem arises from impaired urine concentration mechanisms rather than forced water drinking.

Renal mechanisms for urine concentration

It is obvious that there is a wide range in the normal intake of water, and also in the normal loss of water through the lungs, skin and gut (these three being sources of 'insensible' water loss). Yet despite this, under normal circumstances the osmolality of the plasma is tightly regulated around a mean of 290 mosm/kg, the normal range being within 5 mosm/kg either way. The homeostatic maintenance of this set point for plasma osmolality implies that the kidney is capable of adjusting the rate of water excretion over a wide range, by generating a dilute urine when water is abundant or by generating a concentrated urine when water is scarce. As illustrated in Fig. 3.1, this corresponds in the first case to excretion of urine with an osmolality below 300 (50 mosm/kg being the most dilute urine possible), or in the second case to the production of urine with maximum water extracted (resulting in a typical maximum osmolality around 1200–1400 mosm/kg). We will first look at how the process of concentration is achieved.

In overview, there are two broad requirements for the kidney to be able to produce a urine more concentrated

---

Case 3.1 Water balance and regulation of osmolality: 2

Biochemistry results

The results of Mr Underwood's biochemistry become available the following day. These are shown below:

*Sodium 154 mmol/L
Potassium 4.2 mmol/L
*Chloride 114 mmol/L
Bicarbonate 30 mmol/L
*Urea 11.5 mmol/L
*Creatinine 0.13 mmol/L
Glucose 4.5 mmol/L
*Osmolality 312 mosm/kg

Urine biochemistry

Sodium 26 mmol/L
Glucose 0 mmol/L
Osmolality 80 mosm/kg

The questions now are:

1. What pattern of polyuria is suggested by these results?
2. What further history or investigations are appropriate?

*Results outside the normal range; see Appendix.

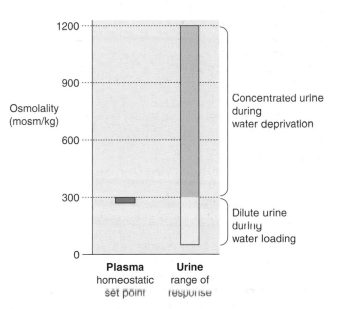

Fig. 3.1 Range of osmolality in plasma and urine.

than the plasma (Fig. 3.2). First, a zone must be created within the renal medulla where the tissue fluid osmolality is high; second, the tubules forming the final segment of the nephron must conduct the urine through this concentrated zone, where water reabsorption can occur passively by osmosis (given that these segments

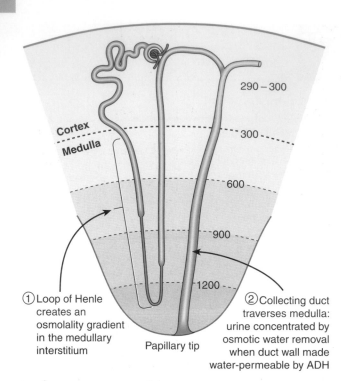

Fig. 3.2 Basic components of the urinary concentrating mechanism. Figures show osmolality of the tissue fluid (in mosm/kg) in different zones of the kidney. The loop of Henle sets up the tissue fluid osmolality gradient within the renal medulla, and the collecting duct traverses this gradient.

can be made permeable to water). The first of these requirements is achieved by the operation of the loop of Henle as it dips into the renal medulla, while the second requirement is fulfilled by the collecting ducts as they pass from the cortex through the medulla on their way to deliver final urine to the renal pelvis. The mechanism whereby the water permeability of the collecting ducts can be increased where appropriate is through the action of circulating vasopressin (antidiuretic hormone; ADH).

Countercurrent multiplication by the loop of Henle

The principle whereby a loop structure can generate a longitudinal gradient of concentration (from the top ends of the loop to its bend) is illustrated in Fig. 3.3. Here the descending and ascending limbs of the loop are shown to be parallel and adjacent, with an intervening layer of tissue fluid lying between them. Flow in the two limbs is said to be countercurrent, in that fluid entering the descending limb (from the end of the proximal tubule) flows downward, while the flow in the adjacent ascending limb is upward, being delivered at the top into the early distal tubule. A second property of the model is that the walls of the descending limb are permeable to water, while those of the ascending limb are impermeable to water. The third and key property of the system is that the walls of the ascending limb contain a pump mechanism capable of removing sodium chloride from

the lumen and adding it to the surrounding interstitial fluid such that a gradient of 200 mosm/kg can be created across the tubular wall at any point. For clarity, the final effect of operating such a system in steady state is built up as a series of discontinuous steps in the diagram.

The flow step shows the effect of introducing some fluid from the proximal tubule into the descending limb (shown with an osmolality of 300 mosm/kg for convenience), and the effect this would have of displacing fluid in the loop in each stage of the model. The second step shows the effect of activating the pump in the ascending limb, creating the 200 mosm/kg gradient across its wall. The third step shows the effect of water movement by osmosis out of the descending limb such that the fluid in that limb attains the same osmolality as the tissue fluid surrounding the ascending limb. It can be seen that the sequential effect of admitting more fluid into the descending limb, and then activating the pump once more, is to multiply the effectiveness of the thick ascending limb's pump mechanism in creating an area of high osmolality around the turn of the loop. In reality, the system operates continuously, resulting in the steady state situation shown in Fig. 3.4.

There are three important consequences of operation of this system. First, the fluid leaving the ascending limb of the loop ends up being quite hypo-osmolar (100 mosm/kg) compared to the fluid entering it. Second, the osmolality near the bend of the loop is raised several fold above the osmolality of the entering fluid. Third, there is ultimately a continuous gradient of tissue osmolality from the 300 mosm/kg pervading near the top of the loop (in the renal cortex) to the 1200 mosm/kg achieved around the turn of the loop of Henle (though not all of this is due to salt accumulation; see below). This provides the environment through which the collecting ducts pass from the cortex through the medulla, providing an opportunity for water extraction from the collecting ducts by osmosis, given that their water permeability is sufficiently high.

From the above model, it can be deduced that three factors would increase the concentrating power achieved by the operation of the loop, namely:

- An increased length of the loop.
- An increased capacity of the pump in the thick ascending limb.
- A reduced flow rate through the loop.

Interesting facts

The role of the loop of Henle in water conservation is illustrated by comparative anatomy and physiology of different mammalian species. In desert-dwelling rodents, such as the marsupial mouse of central Australia, the renal papilla is particularly elongated, containing very long loops of Henle which allow concentration of the urine up to osmolalities greater than 9000 mosmol/kg.

Variations in the length of the loop underlie the differences in the urinary concentrating capacity between different mammalian species, related to the water availability in

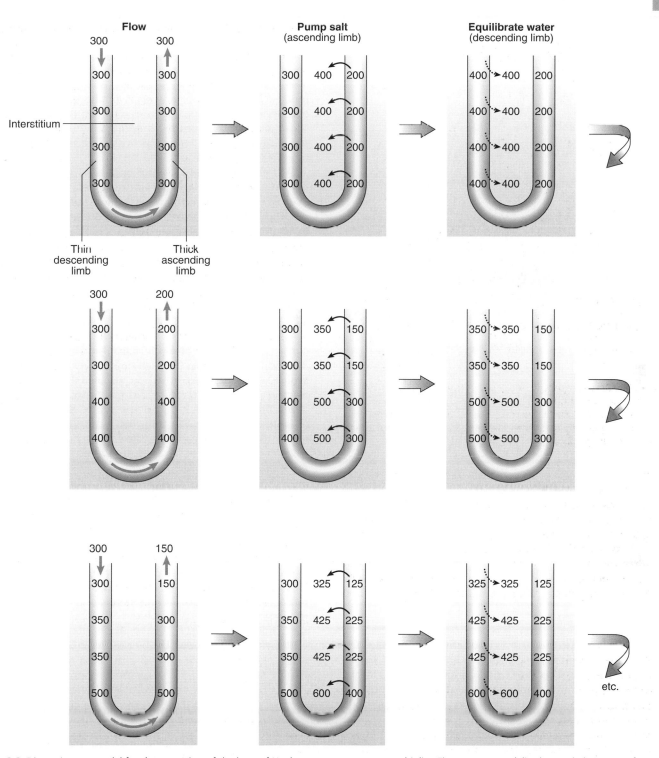

Fig. 3.3 Discontinuous model for the operation of the loop of Henle as a countercurrent multiplier. Figures are osmolality (mosm/kg). See text for detailed description.

the habitat to which they are adapted. Variations in the power of the pump are seen clinically during the action of loop diuretics, such as furosemide (frusemide), which act to inhibit the thick ascending limb's solute reabsorptive capacity. Increases in flow through the loop are seen in volume-expanded states, during which concentrating capacity is reduced.

A number of refinements need to be added to the model to describe the actual situation in the mammalian kidney more fully.

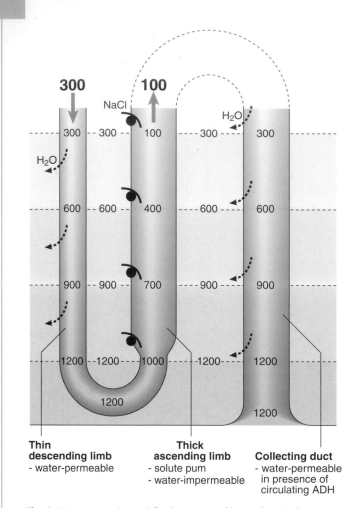

Thin descending limb
- water-permeable

Thick ascending limb
- solute pum
- water-impermeable

Collecting duct
- water-permeable in presence of circulating ADH

Fig. 3.4 Key properties and final outcome of loop of Henle function. The collecting duct properties are those during water deprivation when maximal urine concentration is being achieved. Figures are osmolality (mosm/kg). Note that in the thin descending limb and the collecting duct there is actually a small (5–10 mosm/kg) osmolality gradient between the lumen and the adjacent interstitium (which is higher) to make water move as shown.

First, the osmolality gradient within the medulla is not solely comprised of sodium chloride. Indeed, about half of the interstitial osmolality is contributed by urea. This relatively abundant small organic solute is 'trapped' within the renal medulla because of the different permeability of segments of the nephron to urea (being high in the thin descending and ascending limbs of the loop deep within the medulla, and in the medullary segment of the collecting duct when ADH is present, but low in the thick ascending limb and cortical distal tubule). Thus, under antidiuretic conditions, urea recycles from the medullary collecting duct (out) to the turn of the deep loops of Henle (in), adding to the inner medullary osmolality.

Second, it is clear that a capillary blood supply which crossed the kidney from cortex to medulla would allow for dissipation of the built up solute gradient by diffusion into the capillary blood. This does not occur because of the arrangement of the medullary capillaries themselves

in loops, the vasa recta, which parallel the configuration for the juxtamedullary nephrons. Thus, while medullary solute does enter these vessels in the descending limb, it exits the capillaries in the ascending limb, while water moves in the opposite direction in each case (countercurrent exchange). Since, however, in the steady state the operation of the loop of Henle results in the loss of more solute than water from the tubular lumen, it follows that the vasa recta must remove more solute than water during their passage through the medulla.

A third refinement of the model is that it can be shown that countercurrent multiplication occurs even in the deepest hairpin part of the loop within the inner medulla, before the start of the thick ascending limb. The mechanisms involved here relate to the high water but low sodium permeabilities of the thin descending limb, and the reverse permeabilities of the thin ascending limb.

Action of ADH in the collecting ducts

The second component of the overall process involved in concentrating the urine is the action of ADH, also known as vasopressin (see also *Systems of the Body: The Endocrine System*). This peptide, which is released from the posterior part of the pituitary gland during conditions of water deprivation, acts to increase the water permeability of all segments of the collecting duct, from its earliest parts within the cortex (including the initial segments formed from the late distal tubules) through to the medullary segment as it traverses the outer and inner medulla on the way to emptying at the renal papilla. Thus, when ADH is present in the circulation, water is extensively reabsorbed from the collecting ducts in both the cortex and the medulla. Within the cortex, the maximum osmolality that can be achieved in the luminal fluid corresponds to the 300 mosm/kg present in the interstitial fluid in the cortex. Within the medulla, however, further water abstraction occurs until the osmolality of the urine in the terminal parts of the inner medullary collecting duct can reach the maximum osmolality achieved by the countercurrent mechanism at the tip of the renal papilla, namely about 1200 mosm/kg in man. This reabsorbed water is carried away by the capillaries forming the vasa recta, thus leaving the medullary interstitial osmolality gradient intact.

During states of overhydration, when ADH levels are low (see below), the urine remains dilute, since fluid emerging from the ascending limb of the loop is already hypotonic (see Fig. 3.4). It can be rendered somewhat more dilute by further removal of sodium chloride during passage through the distal tubules and collecting ducts which, under these conditions, are relatively impermeable to water. Hence the urinary osmolality can be lowered from the 100 mosm/kg emerging from the loop to as low as 50 mosm/kg under maximum water diuresis. (In fact, considerable water recovery does occur from the medullary collecting ducts during water diuresis since, although the water permeability is relatively low, the osmolality gradient favouring water reabsorption is high.)

Box 3.1 Conditions required for urinary concentration and dilution

- **To concentrate the urine**
  Adequate solute delivery to the loop of Henle
  Normal function of the loop of Henle
  ADH release into the circulation
  ADH action on the collecting ducts

- **To dilute the urine**
  Adequate solute delivery into the loop of Henle and early distal tubule
  Normal function of the loop of Henle and early distal tubule
  No ADH in the circulation

In summary, Box 3.1 shows in simple form the factors required to achieve concentration of the urine on the one hand, and dilution of the urine on the other. The implications of interfering with these factors for the development of disturbed water balance during clinical conditions is discussed later in this chapter. For the moment it might be noted that loop diuretics clearly have the capacity to impair the kidney's ability to both concentrate and dilute the urine, while the thiazide diuretics, affecting only the component of urinary dilution which occurs in the early distal tubule within the cortex, interfere with maximum dilution of the urine but not with the mechanism for urinary concentration.

Fig. 3.5 Feedback control of plasma osmolality.

Feedback control of plasma osmolality

During conditions of water deprivation, plasma osmolality tends to rise. This osmolality change is detected by specialized neural cells in the hypothalamus called osmoreceptors which, on shrinking, convey electrical signals to adjacent hypothalamic structures, with two parallel outcomes. First, sensation of thirst is stimulated, leading the individual to seek and ingest water actively. Second, cells within the supraoptic and paraventricular hypothalamic nuclei are activated to synthesize ADH, which is transferred bound to a carrier protein neurophysin down specialized axons terminating in the posterior pituitary gland where it is released into the capillary blood. The ADH added to the circulation in this way reaches the kidney, where it acts to increase the water permeability of the collecting duct epithelial cells, resulting in enhanced water reabsorption from the tubular fluid. This, combined with greater intake of water stimulated by thirst, serves to bring the plasma osmolality down towards normal, whereupon osmoreceptor activity reduces and the water-retaining mechanisms are deactivated (Fig. 3.5).

The reverse sequence of events occurs after ingestion of a large volume of water. The plasma is initially diluted slightly as the water is reabsorbed from the gut. This

results in a fall in osmolality which leads the osmoreceptor cells to reduce their activity, following which thirst is suppressed and ADH release is inhibited. These two measures lead to production by the kidney of a dilute urine of high volume, as tubular fluid diluted within the loop of Henle becomes further diluted as it passes through distal nephron segments, which remain impermeable to water in the absence of ADH. As the water load is rapidly excreted, plasma osmolality returns toward normal and baseline conditions are restored.

Figure 3.6 shows the relationship between the plasma osmolality and the concentration of ADH released into the plasma. It can be seen that the threshold for release of ADH is around 280 mosm/kg, only slightly below the normal set point for plasma osmolality (290±5 mosm/kg). A steep linear rise in circulating ADH results as osmolality passes above 290, while ADH release is virtually zero below 280 mosm/kg.

Two factors make the ADH system very effective in the short-term regulation of plasma osmolality. First, ADH is a small peptide (nine amino acids) which has a very short half-life in the circulation, so that its action is not unduly prolonged following its release. Second, the release of ADH from the hypothalamus in response to osmoreceptor signals and its action within the kidney are extremely rapid events, such that the system tracks minute-to-minute

Fig. 3.6 Relationship between plasma osmolality and plasma concentration of ADH.

Fig. 3.7 Cellular mechanism of action of ADH in the collecting duct. AVP, arginine vasopressin (ADH); V2, vasopressin 2 receptor; G, G protein; a.c., adenyl cyclase; PK-A, protein kinase-A; mf, microfilaments; mt, microtubules; AQP2, aquaporin 2.

changes in the osmolality of the plasma, correcting them towards the norm without undue delays.

A variety of non-osmotic stimuli may also cause secretion of ADH, independent of the plasma osmolality. Thus, haemodynamic changes associated with a fall in circulating plasma volume are potent triggers for ADH release. These disturbances are signalled to the brainstem via the volume and pressure sensors located in the central circulation (see Chapter 2), and the result is an independent input into the ADH secretory cells in the hypothalamus, resulting as before in ADH release into the circulation. While stimuli such as hypovolaemia and hypotension can lead to very high levels of ADH in the plasma, the sensitivity of the system to these changes is less than to alterations in plasma osmolality. Thus, while a 1% rise in plasma osmolality is sufficient to trigger a rise in ADH secretion, a 5–10% decrease in blood volume or blood pressure is required to provoke its secretion. Changes of this order do occur, however, in states of circulatory collapse. In addition, other non-osmotic stimuli such as pain, nausea and stress may also provoke ADH release, while alcohol inhibits it.

Mechanism of ADH action in the kidney

Figure 3.7 shows the cellular events involved in the action of ADH in increasing the water permeability of the collecting duct. The ADH in the circulation binds to a specific receptor, named the V2 receptor which is located on the basolateral membrane of the collecting duct epithelial cells. Through an intermediary G protein, this results in the activation of the membrane-bound enzyme adenyl cyclase, which catalyses the conversion of cellular ATP to cyclic AMP. This second messenger is responsible for activating protein kinases within the cytoplasm, which

leads to the phosphorylation of certain proteins involved in the activity of cytoskeletal elements (myofilaments and myofibrils) located in the apical cell cytoplasm. These appear to mobilize vesicles lying below the apical cell membrane which contain preformed water channels comprising the specific channel protein aquaporin 2 (AQP2). Movement of these vesicles into the apical cell membrane results in the addition of AQP2 channels into that membrane, greatly increasing its water permeability. The relatively dilute tubular fluid is now able to move down an osmotic gradient through the cell cytoplasm and into the interstitial fluid and plasma across the basolateral membrane (the water permeability of which is due to the presence of aquaporins 3 and 4).

Two other intrarenal actions of ADH have been defined, both of which amplify its capacity to cause concentration of the urine. First, there is evidence that ADH can increase the activity of the sodium chloride reabsorptive mechanism located in the thick ascending limb of the loop of Henle; and second, ADH increases the permeability of the inner medullary collecting duct to urea. Both of these actions lead to an intensification of the medullary interstitial concentration gradient.

Finally, it is important to mention here that ADH has a separate action, mediated by a different receptor (the V1 receptor, involving intracellular calcium mobilization), by which it promotes vasoconstriction of arterioles throughout the body. This vasoconstrictor action of the hormone increases the blood pressure in the central circulation at the same time as its renal tubular actions serve to retain water. Both actions therefore counteract the circulatory collapse associated with hypovolaemia or dehydration.

Failure to concentrate the urine

We can return now to an analysis of Robert Underwood's apparent failure of urine concentrating capacity. It follows from the above discussion that failure of the normal

Table 3.2 Failure of urinary concentration

Mechanism	Clinical example
Failure to generate medullary concentration gradient:	
Poor solute delivery to the loop of Henle	Low GFR (chronic renal failure)
Impaired action of thick ascending limb of loop	Loop diuretic therapy (furosemide [frusemide])
Failure of ADH effect:	
No ADH released	Central DI (hypothalamic/ pituitary lesion)
No ADH action in kidney	Nephrogenic DI (collecting duct cell dysfunction)
DI, diabetes insipidus; GFR, glomerular filtration rate.	

Fig. 3.8 Urinary omolality *versus* time during a water deprivation test. Characteristic patterns are shown for a normal subject, and for patients with central and nephrogenic diabetes insipidus.

Fig. 3.9 Position of patients with central and nephrogenic diabetes insipidus on the plasma ADH *versus* plasma osmolality graph.

urine concentrating mechanism may result from any of the causes listed in Table 3.2. It is usually quite straightforward to exclude the first causes, involving either established renal failure or the presence of loop diuretics, either of which can lead to inadequate generation of the medullary concentration gradient by the loop of Henle. It is less easy, however, to distinguish whether impaired concentration results from failure to manufacture or release ADH from the brain (hypothalamic or central diabetes insipidus), or from failure of ADH to act appropriately on the renal collecting duct cells (nephrogenic diabetes insipidus).

Both indirect and direct methods for distinguishing between these two conditions are available. First, as shown in Fig. 3.8, a water deprivation test can be performed. In this test, the subject is initially well hydrated such that the urine osmolality is quite low. Urine osmolality is monitored as the patient is observed closely during a period of water deprivation. While the normal subject will develop increased urine osmolality after some 9–12 h of water deprivation as a result of endogenous ADH release, in neither form of diabetes insipidus (DI) will substantial urine concentration occur. Administration of an exogenous dose of ADH at this point will produce a urine concentrating response in the patient with central DI, where there is lack of hypothalamic hormone synthesis, while the patient with nephrogenic DI will have negligible response, reflecting impaired collecting duct capacity to respond to the hormone. Figure 3.9 shows where these two classes of patients would appear on the plasma osmolality *versus* plasma ADH concentration graph. As the plasma osmolality rises, the patient with central DI is unable to raise the near-zero levels of ADH in the plasma appreciably, while the ADH concentration rise in nephrogenic DI may be within the normal range.

The causes of central DI include tumours, trauma, irradiation or cerebrovascular accidents which destroy the relevant regions of the hypothalamus or the pituitary stalk or the posterior pituitary itself. Inflammatory conditions

such as sarcoidosis can occasionally produce the same effect. Causes of nephrogenic DI, on the other hand, include either inherited or acquired problems with the collecting duct ADH response mechanism shown in Fig. 3.7. Inherited conditions have been defined in which there is faulty structure and impaired function of either the V2 receptor protein on the basolateral membrane, or of AQP2 water channels in the apical membrane. Acquired forms of nephrogenic DI can occur when the collecting duct system is affected by infection or obstruction, or where there is interference with the intracellular steps after generation of cyclic AMP, preventing aquaporin translocation into the apical membrane. Examples of this latter mechanism include nephrogenic DI during hypokalaemia, hypercalcaemia and lithium therapy.

Differential diagnosis of hypernatraemia

A useful generalization is that disturbances in ECF sodium *concentration* reflect primary alterations in body water content. In contrast, as discussed in Chapter 2, primary disturbances in body sodium *content* are usually accompanied by parallel changes in the ECF volume status, detected by clinical examination rather than plasma analysis.

When the plasma sodium concentration (and hence osmolality) are increased above normal levels, there is usually a total body water deficit. While this can arise occasionally through inadequate water intake alone, the cause is usually excessive loss of water from the body. As shown in Box 3.2, in some settings this water loss is accompanied by a degree of salt loss, although the water loss in these cases is disproportionately greater. This may occur through the kidney, as for example during diuresis induced by osmotic agents or loop-acting drugs (in water-restricted patients), through the skin (during excessive sweating), or via the gut (during colonic diarrhoea, especially in children).

Water loss unaccompanied by electrolyte depletion does occur in DI, where there is a failure of the normal operation of the ADH system. As described above, this may occur because of hypothalamic failure to synthesize ADH (central DI) or through renal tubular insensitivity to ADH present in the circulation (nephrogenic DI).

Less commonly, hypernatraemia can result from sodium loading, with either normal or reduced body water content. This is an unusual occurrence, and may occur during **enteral** or **parenteral alimentation** with hyperosmotic solutions, or during administration of dietary or therapeutic supplements containing high salt content.

Note that whatever the underlying cause, sustained or severe hypernatraemia must reflect an impaired thirst mechanism, such as that associated with brain damage or stroke, and/or impaired availability of, or access to, water. When thirst mechanisms and water availability are not limiting, the subject will normally drink sufficient water to keep the osmolality from rising very high.

It is clear from the above analysis that the finding of hypernatraemia itself gives no guide as to the total body sodium status. This must be independently assessed using clinical clues, including history and a physical examination seeking signs of hypovolaemia or hypervolaemia (see Chapter 2).

Failure to dilute the urine

The reverse scenario of that described in the previous sections of this chapter occurs when the ECF becomes hypo-osmolar because of impairment of the mechanisms normally involved in excreting excess ingested water; that is, in diluting the urine. As summarized in Box 3.1, this process requires adequate delivery of filtrate through the segments of the nephron capable of lowering the osmolality

---

Case 3.1

Water balance and regulation of osmolality: 3

The diagnosis

Mr Underwood's history, physical examination and biochemical results were reviewed, looking for clues to one of the known mechanisms for impaired urinary concentration. Severe renal impairment was excluded by the virtually normal plasma creatinine concentration, and loop diuretics had never been prescribed or taken by the patient.

Initially, investigations were directed towards excluding the possibility of hypothalamic DI by arranging for an assay of plasma ADH level at a time when the patient was dehydrated and hyperosmolar, as at presentation. A cerebral CT scan was also organized, looking for evidence of structural damage in the area of the hypothalamus or pituitary fossa.

At this point, however, the patient volunteered that he had been receiving psychiatric treatment for 1 month, following his presentation in an agitated and hypomanic state. He had started on lithium carbonate tablets, 500 mg bd, and therapy was currently being stabilized in conjunction with his psychiatrist. Indeed, a plasma lithium concentration of 0.9 mmol/L had recently been obtained by his psychiatrist, with whom contact was now made.

A diagnosis of lithium-induced nephrogenic DI was therefore made. Consistent with this, the plasma ADH concentration result later came back in the high normal range, appropriate for the elevated plasma osmolality. The cerebral CT scan proved to be normal.

In this situation, management consists of several steps: the patient was advised always to maintain an adequate water intake, but not to drink more than thirst demanded. If indeed the psychiatric judgement was that lithium therapy should be continued, given its efficacy in controlling the mood swings of **bipolar affective disorder**, close monitoring of the resultant plasma lithium levels was recommended to maintain the serum lithium within and at the lower end of the recommended therapeutic range (0.4–0.8 mmol/L). Finally, if polyuria and thirst persisted and were troublesome to the patient, a trial of amiloride therapy could be considered. Experimental and clinical evidence suggests that this agent blocks uptake of lithium as well as sodium through the apical cation channel in the cortical collecting duct, mitigating the extent of lithium's interference with the intracellular steps in ADH.

---

of the luminal fluid by removing sodium while remaining impermeable to water. These properties are possessed by the ascending limb of the loop of Henle and the early (convoluted) part of the distal tubule. Secondly, ADH secretion must be suppressed appropriately by the low plasma osmolality so that water is not reabsorbed from the collecting duct system.

In assessing the patient with inappropriate water retention, it is thus necessary first to rule out renal failure

Box 3.2 Differential diagnosis of hypernatraemia

- **Water deficit with proportionately smaller sodium deficit**
  Renal: osmotic or loop diuretic (during water restriction)
  Extrarenal: skin (excessive sweating); gut (colonic diarrhoea)

- **Water deficit alone**
  Renal: central or nephrogenic diabetes insipidus

- **Sodium loading with normal or reduced body water**
  Enteral or parenteral alimentation
  Intravenous or oral salt administration

Note that in all cases there is usually some blunting of the normal thirst mechanism and/or restricted access to water.

Box 3.3 Differential diagnosis of hyponatraemia*

- **Sodium deficit with relative water retention**
  Renal: thiazides and loop diuretics (during water drinking), adrenocortical failure
  Extrarenal: gut (e.g. vomiting)

- **Water retention alone**
  SIADH: ectopic ADH secretion from tumour, lung disease, CNS disease, drugs
  Hypothyroidism

- **Sodium retention with relatively greater water retention**
  Generalized oedema states: congestive cardiac failure, cirrhosis, nephrotic syndrome
  Chronic kidney disease

*Note that psychogenic polydipsia and other forms of forced water drinking are excluded from this table. SIADH, syndrome of inappropriate ADH secretion.

(low GFR); second, to exclude use of diuretic drugs acting on the thick ascending limb (e.g. furosemide; frusemide) or the early distal tubule (e.g. thiazides); and third, to determine that ADH is not being released into the circulation. In regard to the latter, it must be remembered that ADH release can be triggered not only by a rise in plasma osmolality, but also by non-osmotic stimuli such as hypovolaemia, hypotension, nausea, stress and pain. Sometimes these stimuli are present without elevation of the plasma osmolality, resulting in water retention sufficient to drive the plasma osmolality below the normal range.

Differential diagnosis of hyponatraemia

These considerations are most commonly brought to bear in assessing the clinical problem of hyponatraemia. Nearly all of the hyponatraemic states are associated with sustained action of ADH in retaining water from the collecting ducts, despite the presence of hypo-osmolality which would otherwise be expected to switch off ADH release. The main exception is forced water drinking, such as that which occurs in psychogenic polydipsia: in this situation the primary excess of ingested water, and slight expansion of ECF volume, both act to switch off ADH, such that maximal urine dilution occurs. Hyponatraemia only develops to the extent that water ingestion continues at a rate exceeding its maximal excretion rate through the kidney.

The other causes of hyponatraemia are summarized in Box 3.3. Relative water retention may occur in conditions where there is a sodium deficit and hypovolaemia. This is due most commonly to sodium losses through the gastrointestinal tract (e.g. vomiting) or via the kidney (e.g. during diuretic action). As previously mentioned, in the case of loop and early distal acting diuretics, sodium loss is compounded by interference with the mechanisms for generating dilute urine in these nephron segments.

Deficiency of **adrenocortical hormones** also results in renal sodium wasting. In all of these conditions, ADH is activated through the mechanism of hypovolaemia consequent upon ECF volume reduction. The stage is thus set for persistence of hyponatraemia until the sodium deficit is restored.

Water retention without a major change in body sodium can occur where ADH levels are elevated with neither an osmotic nor a hypovolaemic stimulus. In the syndrome of inappropriate ADH secretion (SIADH), ADH is released into the circulation either from an ectopic site, such as a hormone-secreting tumour (e.g. lung cancer), or from the posterior pituitary, secondary to non-malignant lung disease which may stimulate intrathoracic receptors so as to mimic volume depletion. A variety of drugs may also stimulate central ADH release, e.g. phenothiazines, vincristine, cyclophosphamide. In SIADH, there is hyponatraemia with plasma hypo-osmolality, but with a urine which remains inappropriately concentrated, i.e. not maximally dilute. The urine sodium concentration is relatively high, which excludes plasma volume contraction in which it would be low.

A final category of hyponatraemia is that which arises when there is salt retention, but relatively greater water retention. This can occur during any of the conditions causing systemic oedema, such as congestive cardiac failure, nephrotic syndrome and cirrhosis. The water retention in these cases is partly because of the impaired GFR and avid proximal sodium and water reabsorption, which limit delivery of solute through the diluting segments of the nephron, and partly because of ADH release into the circulation. ADH secretion in these conditions is triggered by a reduction in the 'effective' arterial blood volume related to the impaired haemodynamics prevailing in each condition (see also Chapter 6).

The management of hyponatraemia depends first on defining the aetiology and reversing the causative condition wherever possible. This being done, treatment for hypovol-aemic states involves volume replacement with intravenous sodium chloride infusions. For hypervolaemic conditions, sodium restriction accompanied by even tighter water restriction is necessary. In SIADH and related conditions, restriction of water alone is the mainstay of treatment.

Interesting facts

In the treatment of hyponatraemia, it is critically impor-tant to relate the rate of correction to the rate of devel-opment of the disorder. Unduly slow correction of acute hyponatraemia can lead to death from cerebral oedema as water enters cerebral neurons and causes brain com-pression. On the other hand, overly rapid correction of chronic hyponatraemia can lead to death from demyelina-tion of cerebral neurons which undergo osmotic shrinkage and separation from their myelin sheaths.

Again it is worth reiterating that a low plasma sodium concentration generally reflects the relative excess of water in the ECF, and gives no reliable guide to the total body sodium and volume status. This must be deter-mined from the history and by physical examination, using guidelines provided in Chapter 2.

ACID–BASE BALANCE AND REGULATION OF pH

4

Chapter objectives

After studying this chapter you should be able to:

1. Define the normal range for plasma pH.

2. Explain the role of the kidney in the steady state elimination of acid produced daily by metabolism.

3. Outline the defence mechanisms which act to prevent an abrupt change in pH in response to an acid load.

4. Describe the mechanism for acid transport in the different nephron segments.

5. Recognize the clinical and biochemical features of metabolic acidosis, list some causes and give an approach to the differential diagnosis.

6. Recognize metabolic alkalosis, list some causes, and explain the pathophysiology of this disturbance during prolonged vomiting.

Introduction

Just as the kidney is a critical organ in defending the normal set points for extracellular fluid (ECF) volume, osmolality and potassium concentration, it also plays a central role in the homeostasis of the plasma pH. While chemical buffering mechanisms and respiratory elimination of carbon dioxide are important in immediate responses to disturbances in acid–base balance, it falls to the kidney to make long-term adjustments in the rate of acid excretion which allows the external balance with respect to hydrogen ion concentration to be maintained. This chapter will focus on the mechanisms whereby the kidney achieves this role, and the origin of some disturbances of this system in disease. See Case 4.1:1.

The clue in this case that there is a disturbance of acid–base metabolism is that the bicarbonate concentration, representing the base component of the principal

Case
4.1

Acid–base balance and regulation of pH: 1

A case of acidosis

Mrs Mary Loy is a 48-year-old woman of Chinese background who has been sent by her family doctor to the Emergency Department because of his concern about her clinical condition and some biochemical results.

She had been complaining for some weeks of increasing lethargy, an extensive rash and 'heavy breathing'. She had been receiving treatment for 4 years for systemic lupus erythematosus (SLE), a multiorgan autoimmune condition for which a consultant rheumatologist had prescribed prednisone. However, Mrs Loy confessed to having discontinued this medication some 10 months earlier because she was unhappy about its side effects.

On examination she was febrile, unwell and had an erythematous rash on her face and limbs. Her blood pressure was 110/80, pulse rate 100 beats/min and respiratory rate 20/min, the breathing being deep and sighing. The referring doctor's letter indicated that he had obtained a urinalysis result that morning showing: pH 7, blood and protein.

He had also obtained plasma biochemistry the previous day, the results of which are as follows:

Sodium 135 mmol/L
*Potassium 3.1 mmol/L
*Chloride 113 mmol/L
*Bicarbonate 13 mmol/L
Urea 8.0 mmol/L
Creatinine 0.09 mmol/L

The family doctor is particularly concerned about the low bicarbonate, which he interprets as a sign of acid build-up, and seeks full evaluation of her clinical and metabolic problem.

*Results outside the normal range; see Appendix.

physiological buffer system, is greatly reduced below the normal range. This is consistent with acid accumulation in the ECF, for which we must explore both the cause and the consequences.

The key parameter involved in acid–base regulation is the concentration of H in the ECF. The physiological set point for this parameter is 40 nmol/L, usually expressed (using the negative base 10 logarithm) as the pH, which is normally 7.40. So important is homeostasis of this parameter to the normal operation of metabolism and cellular function that pH is tightly regulated in the range 7.38–7.42, although a somewhat wider range is compatible with life (7.0–7.8).

Two forms of acid are generated as a result of normal metabolic processes. Oxidative metabolism produces a large amount of CO_2 daily, and this so-called 'volatile acid' is excreted through the lungs. Carbon dioxide effectively acts as an acid in body fluids because of the following reactions:

$$CO_2 + H_2O \xrightleftharpoons{\text{c.a.}} H_2CO_3 \rightleftharpoons H^+ + HCO_3^-$$

The first reaction (formation of carbonic acid, H_2CO_3) is the rate-limiting step and is normally slow, but in the presence of the enzyme carbonic anhydrase (c.a.) the reaction is greatly accelerated. The subsequent ionization of carbonic acid proceeds almost instantaneously. This equation can be rearranged to enhance its physiological utility in the form shown in Fig. 4.1, as the Henderson–Hasselbalch equation.

The other form of acid, the so-called 'non-volatile acid', results from the metabolism of dietary protein, resulting in the accumulation of some 70 mmol of acid per day in an average adult on a typical western meat-containing diet.

The most important mechanism preventing change in the pH of the ECF is the carbonic acid/bicarbonate buffer system outlined above. The importance of this buffer pair relates to certain key properties: bicarbonate is present in

$$pH = 6.1 + \log \frac{[HCO_3^-]}{0.03 \times pCO_2}$$

Fig. 4.1 Effect of changes in HCO_3^- and pCO_2 on net pH of the plasma. This is an applied version of the Henderson–Hasselbalch equation. Normal plasma $[HCO_3^-]$ = 24 mmol/L, normal pCO_2 = 40 mm Hg, giving a normal plasma pH of 7.40. The pH will return to 7.40 as long as the ratio of $[HCO_3]:[0.03 \times pCO_2]$ is 20:1. *Note that changes in HCO_3 concentration are also made as part of the renal correction of sustained *metabolic* acid–base disturbances as long as the kidney itself is not the cause of the primary disturbance.

a relatively high concentration in the ECF (24 mmol/L) and the components of the buffer system are effectively under physiological control: the CO_2 by the lungs, and the bicarbonate by the kidneys. These relationships are illustrated in Fig. 4.1.

It is clear from this relationship that a shift in pH can be brought about by either a primary change in the bicarbonate concentration (metabolic disturbances) or in the partial pressure of CO_2 in the blood (respiratory disturbances). However, it can also be seen that alterations in each of these parameters may represent a compensatory change whereby either the kidney or the lung can act to limit the extent of pH change which would occur because of a primary disturbance in respiratory function or in metabolism, respectively. The patterns of resulting clinical acid–base disturbances will be discussed later in this chapter.

Role of the kidney in H$^+$ balance

Before we can make further progress in analysing the acid–base problem in our patient, it is necessary to consider the role the kidney plays in maintaining acid–base balance under normal conditions. Given that bicarbonate buffer is freely filtered at the glomerulus and that there is a daily load of non-volatile acid to be excreted into the urine, there must be two components to the nephron's task: reabsorption of filtered bicarbonate, and addition of net acid to the tubular fluid.

Bicarbonate reabsorption

Bicarbonate is the principal physiological buffer in the plasma and it is freely filtered at the glomerulus. If this bicarbonate were not fully reabsorbed by the tubular system, there would be ongoing losses of essential buffer into the urine, resulting in progressive acidification of the body fluids as metabolic acid production continued. In fact, bicarbonate excretion is essentially zero under normal conditions because of the extensive and efficient reabsorption of bicarbonate, principally in the proximal tubule as shown in Fig. 4.2.

Fig. 4.2 Mechanism of proximal tubular bicarbonate reabsorption. c.a., carbonic anhydrase.

As discussed in Chapter 2, the cells in this tubular segment contain a sodium–hydrogen exchange carrier molecule known as NHE-3 in the apical cell membrane. As sodium enters the cell from the luminal fluid down its electrochemical gradient via this carrier, it effectively removes hydrogen ions from the cell cytoplasm and adds them to the luminal fluid. The hydrogen ions are generated within the cell by the action of the enzyme carbonic anhydrase, which catalyses the reaction between CO_2 and water to produce carbonic acid. This rapidly breaks down to produce the hydrogen ions that are secreted into the lumen, and bicarbonate ions which are cotransported on a carrier with sodium (probably in a ratio $3HCO_3^-:1Na^+$) across the basolateral cell membrane into the plasma. (Note that this is equivalent to saying that the dissociation of cellular water yields a hydrogen ion and a hydroxyl ion, which reacts with cytoplasmic CO_2 under the influence of carbonic anhydrase to produce the bicarbonate for basolateral extrusion.) Carbonic anhydrase also exists on the brush border membrane on the luminal surface of these cells. Here it catalyses the breakdown of carbonic acid formed as the secreted hydrogen ion reacts with filtered bicarbonate, releasing water and CO_2 which passes freely across the cell membrane, allowing the cycle to repeat.

The net outcome of this process is that the filtered sodium bicarbonate passing through the proximal tubule is effectively reabsorbed, although the bicarbonate added to the plasma in a given turn of the cycle is not the same one appearing in the lumen with sodium. This process accounts for reabsorption of some 85% of filtered bicarbonate, and operates at a high capacity but generates a low gradient of hydrogen ion concentration across the epithelium, with the luminal pH falling only slightly from 7.4 at the glomerulus to around 7.0 at the end of the proximal tubule. This is both because of the presence of carbonic anhydrase in the luminal compartment and because the epithelium is 'leaky' to hydrogen ions.

Net acid excretion

It is important to understand that the process described above has not done anything to remove net acid from the body, since the fate of the secreted H$^+$ in this segment is effectively to conserve most of the filtered bicarbonate. Under circumstances requiring removal of net acid from the body, the tubules must still carry out two more steps.

- Secrete further acid into the tubular lumen beyond that needed to reabsorb all filtered bicarbonate.

- Provide a buffer in the tubular fluid to assist in the removal of this acid (this is necessary since the maximum acidification which can be achieved in the lumen – around pH 4.5 – would not allow for excretion of the metabolic acid load needing elimination).

These two requirements are fulfilled in more distal nephron segments. As shown in Figs 4.3 and 4.4, acid is secreted into the lumen of the late distal tubule and collecting ducts by an H$^+$-ATPase located in the apical cell membrane.

Fig. 4.3 Titration of filtered buffer (phosphate) by acid secreted in the distal nephron. Movements of filtered sodium ions are not shown. c.a., carbonic anhydrase.

Fig. 4.4 Titration of manufactured buffer (ammonia) by acid secreted in the distal nephron. Ammonia is largely synthesized in proximal tubular cells and reaches the distal tubular lumen by gaseous diffusion from the blood. c.a., carbonic anhydrase.

This pump has been found in the intercalated cells within the cortical collecting duct and in the apical membrane of the outer medullary collecting duct cells. The H^+ undergoing secretion in this way is generated within the tubular cells by a reaction facilitated by carbonic anhydrase, as described for the proximal tubule. Again, the bicarbonate generated within the cell by this process passes across the basolateral membrane, this time via a chloride–bicarbonate exchange carrier (anion exchanger 1), into the plasma. However, here the bicarbonate does not replace a filtered bicarbonate molecule, but represents a 'new' bicarbonate, effectively counteracting the consumption of buffer which would have occurred had the excreted acid been retained in the body.

Two types of buffer are involved in excretion of this net acid. The glomerular filtrate contains a limited amount of non-bicarbonate buffer which is capable of taking up some of the H^+, as shown in Fig. 4.3. The main molecule involved is monohydrogen phosphate HPO_4^{2-} which is titrated in the distal lumen to dihydrogen phosphate (HPO_4^-) which is excreted in the urine with sodium. This reaction has limited capacity (removing

up to 30 mmol of H^+/day) and tends to proceed as the urine pH falls along the distal nephron segments, typically from 7 down to 6 and below, the pK (acid dissociation constant) of this buffer system being 6.8. This form of excreted H^+ is sometimes called 'titratable acid' as it can be quantitated by back-titrating a specimen of urine.

The other form of buffer involved in removal of secreted acid is that manufactured by the kidney itself, namely ammonia (NH_3). Renal tubular cells, especially those of the proximal tubule, contain the enzyme glutaminase, which catalyses the production of NH_3 from the nitrogen-rich amino acid glutamine. Ammonia itself is a lipid-soluble gas, which diffuses freely through the kidney tissue and is converted to its protonated form ammonium (NH_4) in acidic environments (it is also concentrated in the renal medulla by recirculation in the loop of Henle). As the luminal pH falls from the proximal to the distal nephron segments, the NH_4^+ becomes increasingly 'trapped' in the luminal fluid compartment where it is washed away into the urine, associated with chloride ions. Again this constitutes removal of an unwanted H^+ from the body, with restoration of a 'new' bicarbonate molecule to the ECF. The importance of this mechanism for acid excretion is that it is linked to an abundant and regulated source of buffer production (NH_3) of essentially unlimited capacity. Thus, under conditions of acid build-up (especially chronic acidosis), NH_3 synthesis is stimulated and acid excretion (as ammonium) is greatly increased, allowing systemic acid–base balance to be maintained.

Note that despite the action of NH_3 to buffer the build-up of free acid in the late segments of the nephron, the pH of the tubular fluid does fall along the collecting duct system, resulting in final urinary pH as low as 4.5. This occurs both because the distal nephron is relatively impermeable to H^+ and because there is no carbonic anhydrase in the luminal compartment in these tubular segments. This means that the dehydration of carbonic acid formed in the lumen is slow, allowing H^+ to accumulate.

In summary, under conditions of normal dietary protein consumption, a slightly alkaline plasma pH of 7.40 is maintained despite the generation of about 70 mmol of hydrogen ion (as non-volatile acid) per day. The kidney's role in maintaining this pH homeostasis is achieved by generating an acidic urine in which the net daily excess of acid can be removed. It does this in the following ways.

- Reabsorbing all bicarbonate buffer filtered into the urine.
- Secreting H^+ for excretion with filtered buffers such as phosphate.
- Secreting H^+ for excretion with the manufactured buffer ammonia.

Disturbances of acid–base balance: acidosis

Following from the above principles, we can now examine how the kidney is involved in the response to acid–base disturbances, and will consider first the situation of

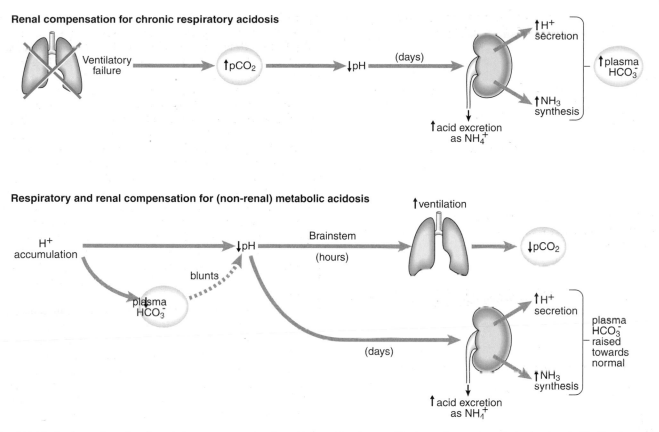

Fig. 4.5 Mechanisms of renal and respiratory compensation for acid–base disturbances. The immediate action of physicochemical buffers is omitted for clarity.

excess acid accumulation, or acidosis. This may arise as a result of either of two primary disturbances.

Respiratory acidosis

Respiratory acidosis results from the accumulation of CO_2 in the body as a result of failure of pulmonary ventilation. This itself may occur after lesions either in the central nervous system (e.g. depression of cerebral function, spinal cord injury) or in peripheral nervous pathways involved in ventilating the lungs (peripheral nerve and muscle disorders), or in some forms of lung disease involving impaired gas diffusion (refer also to *Systems of the Body: The Respiratory System*).

The decrease in body fluid pH resulting from carbonic acid generation is initially buffered to a limited extent by the reaction of carbonic acid with intracellular buffers such as haemoglobin, leading to the release of small amounts of bicarbonate into the plasma. However, longer term restoration of body fluid pH balance requires the excretion by the kidney of the net acid retained during the period of hypoventilation.

This is achieved by the three steps described above, namely total reabsorption of filtered bicarbonate, titration of all available filtered buffers, and increased generation of ammonia within the kidney to allow for a higher-than-baseline level of net acid excretion as ammonium ion.

This latter step is stimulated both by intracellular acidosis and by the elevated pCO_2 which is associated with respiratory acidosis. Over a few days, a new steady state is achieved in which renal excretion of net acid matches that being retained by the lungs, the urine pH being low and the plasma bicarbonate being raised above baseline values (Fig. 4.5).

Metabolic acidosis

Metabolic acidosis (or, more correctly, non-respiratory acidosis), on the other hand, is associated with the accumulation of non-volatile acid within the body. There are essentially three components to the protective response which limits the fall in pH which would otherwise occur.

Physicochemical buffering

The first defence against a fall in the pH of the body fluids after addition of an acid load is the buffering of H^+ by available bases, particularly bicarbonate which is abundant in the ECF. This results in a fall in the plasma bicarbonate, and hence a lesser fall in the plasma pH than would otherwise have occurred. A variety of extracellular and intracellular proteins provide a further reserve of H^+ binding sites, and a limited amount of tissue phosphate also contributes some buffer capacity. These reactions are essentially complete within a few minutes of addition of acid to the body fluids, though further buffering occurs in bone and other tissues over the ensuing hours and days.

Respiratory response

Despite initial buffering, the pH of the plasma will still fall somewhat during acidosis, and this acts as a potent stimulus to increase the ventilation rate via the activation of chemoreceptors within the brainstem (ventral medulla) which respond to a fall in pH of the cerebrospinal fluid. Clinically this manifests as a deep, rapid breathing pattern (Kussmaul respiration). Over a matter of minutes to hours, this response drives the CO_2 below normal, and thus serves to blunt the fall in ECF pH by shifting the carbonic acid equilibrium reaction (see Fig. 4.1). This respiratory response provides a medium-term compensation for the acidosis produced by the metabolic disturbance. Note that while the resulting plasma pH is brought up towards 7.40, it is not fully normalized, and never 'overshoots', as a result of respiratory compensation alone.

Renal response

Steady state correction of the acid–base disturbance requires the development over several days of an increased capacity by the kidney to excrete the metabolic acid load. This involves reabsorption of all filtered bicarbonate, maximum titration of filtered buffers with secreted H^+, and increased intrarenal synthesis of ammonia, which combines with secreted hydrogen ions in the luminal compartment and appears in the urine as large quantities of ammonium. The urine pH falls to minimum levels (around 4.5) and the plasma bicarbonate, lowered initially by the reaction with added acid and subsequently by the hyperventilation response, is elevated back up into the normal range. The net result is a restoration of plasma pH to normal.

Before leaving the subject of renal acid secretion, a number of factors which have been identified as regulators of this process should be listed. The principal factors causing an increase in H^+ secretion by the nephron include:

- increase in filtered load of bicarbonate
- decrease in ECF volume
- decrease in plasma pH
- increase in blood pCO_2
- hypokalaemia
- aldosterone.

Note that the first two factors listed result in increased proximal bicarbonate reabsorption, while the later factors act in distal nephron segments to enhance net acid excretion. The common mediator in the case of the last four factors is probably a decrease in the intracellular pH of the tubular cells, which not only activates the hydrogen ion secretory mechanism but also enhances tubular ammonia synthesis. See Case 4.1:2.

Case 4.1 Acid–base balance and regulation of pH: 2

The arterial blood gases

Returning to the case of Mrs Loy, crucial early data needed to clarify her acid–base status are the pH and pCO_2 of the arterial blood. These are obtained immediately after her admission to hospital, and give the following results:

pH 7.37
*pCO_2 22 mmHg
*$HCO3^-$ 13 mmol/L
pO_2 103 mm Hg

These data confirm that her problem is primarily an acidosis (pH < 7.40) of metabolic origin (low HCO_3^-) which has undergone a considerable degree of respiratory compensation (low pCO_2). However, the presence of the low bicarbonate concentration implies that the kidney has not achieved long-term correction of the underlying acid accumulation.

The question now arises: what is the source of the metabolic acid load that is playing a major part in this presentation?

Before completing an analysis of her acid–base problem, we might take note of one clue present in the data available already. Whatever the cause of metabolic acid build-up, there is some problem with kidney function in this case since urinalysis showed a pH of 7. According to the description above of an expected renal response to acidosis involving excretion of a maximally acidic urine (pH < 5), the urine pH in this case is quite inappropriate and would appear to point to a primary problem located within the kidney itself. As will be seen, this was indeed the case.

Patterns of metabolic acidosis

Two basic types of metabolic acidosis can be distinguished, on the basis of the effect they have on readily measurable plasma parameters. In one type, acid might be added as hydrochloric (mineral) acid, or there might be a primary loss of bicarbonate buffer from the ECF. In this pattern, there is no addition to the plasma of a new acid anion. In the second type, the accumulating acid might be in the form of an organic acid where the acid anion accumulates in the plasma to replace the falling bicarbonate.

These concepts are shown in diagrammatic form in Fig. 4.6. When the concentrations of the commonly measured cations in the blood (sodium and potassium) are added, there is in normal plasma an apparent discrepancy of some 15 mmol/L over and above the sum of the two commonly measured anions (chloride and bicarbonate). This 'anion gap' is largely explained by the multiple negative charges on plasma protein molecules. It can be seen that, where mineral acid is added or bicarbonate is lost (pattern A), the fall in plasma bicarbonate is

Fig. 4.6 Patterns of metabolic acidosis. All figures are in mmol/L. AG, anion gap.

compensated by a rise in chloride, resulting in no change in the apparent anion gap. In pattern B, however, the bicarbonate may fall to the same extent, but this is accounted for by the addition of the organic acid anion, which, being itself unmeasured, adds to the apparent anion gap, and the plasma chloride does not change from normal. This simple analysis provides an initial tool for the diagnosis of the cause of a metabolic acidosis, where this is not obvious.

Some causes of normal anion gap metabolic acidosis are given in Table 4.1. Rarely, the cause is addition of hydrochloric acid or ammonium chloride, usually in a setting of medical investigation or treatment. More commonly, there is a problem either in the gastrointestinal tract involving loss of bicarbonate from the lower bowel, or in the kidney. In the latter case, the normal mechanisms for H$^+$ secretion into the lumen of the nephron may be impaired, either in the proximal tubule (such as by the carbonic anhydrase inhibitor acetazolamide), or in the distal nephron (where the processes involved in urinary acidification are defective). As a group, these disorders of renal acid excretion are called renal tubular acidoses, and will be discussed further later in this chapter.

Causes of the increased anion gap pattern of metabolic acidosis are given in Table 4.2. The organic acid load in these conditions may be classified as to whether it is of endogenous or exogenous origin. In some cases, when specifically suspected, such as lactate in lactic acidosis,

the organic acid anion can be measured in the blood. In other cases, however, the clinical history provides a strong clue as to the cause, e.g. the accumulation of ketoacids in diabetic ketoacidosis, or of salicylate following aspirin intoxication (this latter disorder being complicated by respiratory alkalosis because of ventilatory stimulation). Of note is the predisposition of alcoholic patients to a number of forms of increased anion gap metabolic acidosis. These include starvation ketosis, lactic acidosis and intoxication by methanol or ethylene glycol (when consumed as alternatives to alcohol). Where metabolic acidosis is associated with advanced renal failure, the cause is usually the accumulation of complex organic acids normally excreted by filtration and proximal tubular secretion, and the result is an increased anion gap. See Case 4.1:3.

Renal tubular acidosis

Metabolic acidosis can arise as a result of failure of renal tubular segments to secrete hydrogen ions in the absence of any major impairment of glomerular filtration rate. This acidosis of renal tubular origin is not associated with accumulation of any organic acid anion, and so the anion gap remains normal. Two basic variants of the condition, which can be either congenital or acquired, are described.

Case 4.1 Acid–base balance and regulation of pH: 3

The diagnosis

Mrs Loy's electrolyte profile was examined and an anion gap of 12 mmol/L was calculated (see original biochemistry data). There was no history of gastrointestinal disturbance and the urine pH was noted to be inappropriately high at 7. An interim diagnosis of renal tubular acidosis was made.

Further investigation, directed toward defining the immunological activity of her underlying connective tissue disease, revealed that the levels of **antinuclear antibodies** (including antibodies to double-stranded DNA) were elevated, and serum **complement** levels were low, consistent with activated SLE. In addition, the urine contained many red cells and red cell casts (see Chapter 7), and a large amount of protein. Renal biopsy confirmed severe diffuse inflammation affecting the glomeruli as well as the **tubulointerstitium**.

A diagnosis of reactivated SLE was made, with the complications of diffuse lupus nephritis (see Chapter 7) and renal tubular acidosis. The distal tubular dysfunction in this setting reflects a disruptive effect of the interstitial inflammatory changes on the transport properties of the tubules.

Table 4.1 Causes of normal anion gap metabolic acidosis

Disorder	Mechanism
Inorganic acid addition:	
Infusion/ingestion of HCl, NH$_4$Cl	Exogenous acid load
Gastrointestinal base loss:	
*Diarrhoea	Loss of bicarbonate from gut
Small bowel fistula/drainage	Loss of bicarbonate from gut
Surgical diversion of urine into gut loops	Secretion of KHCO$_3$ by bowel mucosa
Renal base loss/acid retention:	
Proximal renal tubular acidosis	Renal tubular bicarbonate wasting
Distal renal tubular acidosis	Impaired renal tubular acid secretion

*Diarrhoea alone is rarely associated with marked acidosis unless it is severe and prolonged.

Table 4.2 Causes of increased anion gap metabolic acidosis

Disorder	Anion(s)	Clues to diagnosis
Endogenous acid load:		
Diabetic ketoacidosis	Acetoacetate, beta-OH butyrate	Hyperglycaemia, ketonuria
Starvation ketosis	Acetoacetate, beta-OH butyrate	Hypoglycaemia
Lactic acidosis	Lactate	Shock, hypoxia, liver disease
Renal failure	Organic acids	Reduced glomerular filtration rate
Exogenous acid load:		
Salicylate poisoning	Salicylate	Associated with respiratory alkalosis
Methanol poisoning	Formate	Visual complaints, often alcoholic
Ethylene glycol poisoning	Glycolate, oxalate	Oxalate crystalluria, often alcoholic

- In proximal renal tubular acidosis (RTA), the defect lies in the mechanism normally present within the proximal tubular epithelium for reabsorbing bicarbonate (refer to Fig. 4.2). Thus, either because of a specific defect in one of the components of the cellular acid secretory mechanism in this segment or because of non-specific damage to, or malfunction of, the proximal tubular epithelium as a whole, filtered bicarbonate is incompletely reabsorbed. This results in a large flow of bicarbonate, together with sodium, through later nephron segments. Plasma bicarbonate falls, blood pH falls, and bicarbonate appears in the urine.

- In distal RTA, the defect is in the late distal tubule and collecting duct segments, where acid secretion is mediated by an H$^+$-ATPase. In inherited ('classical') forms of this disorder, the defect is either in the hydrogen pump itself or in the anion exchanger in the basolateral membrane (see Fig. 4.7). In other forms, such as that induced by amphotericin (an antifungal antibiotic), the impairment of net acid secretion results from back-leak of hydrogen ions across an epithelium which is made abnormally permeable to these ions.

Some causes of proximal and distal RTA are given in Box 4.1. Both proximal and distal RTA may be inherited as a primary defect, but a number of other conditions may produce secondary RTA in either segment. Notably, an alteration in proximal tubular function can be induced by high **paraprotein** levels as in **myeloma**, or by the carbonic anhydrase inhibitor acetazolamide. Distal RTA, on the other hand, can be caused by conditions associated with polyclonal **hyperglobulinaemia**, including SLE, as in the patient studied in this chapter (see also *Systems of the Body: The Musculoskeletal System*). Other forms of structural tubulointerstitial disease can produce the same defect, and a number of drugs and toxins are also prone to damage this segment selectively.

Apart from the differences in clinical setting and aetiology between the proximal and distal types of RTA, a number of physiological differences exist. In the distal form, the impaired operation of the collecting duct H$^+$

Fig. 4.7 Sites of defect in two variants of distal renal tubular acidosis (RTA).

pump means that, no matter how severe the systemic acidosis, the urine pH can never be lowered appropriately, and generally remains above 5.5. Bicarbonate loss is not prominent since proximal reabsorption is generally intact. However, in early or mild forms of proximal RTA there is considerable leak of bicarbonate into the urine, which again has an inappropriately high pH since the distal segments are unable to acidify the urine as long as large amounts of bicarbonate are flooding through the lumen from the proximal segments. However, when acidosis is more severe in proximal RTA, the plasma bicarbonate falls because of buffering of the accumulated acid. As a result, a point may be reached where the reduced filtered amount of bicarbonate can be largely reabsorbed by the defective proximal tubular reabsorptive mechanism. The intact distal segments can then reabsorb a small distal leak of bicarbonate, as normally occurs. In this situation the distal tubular secretory pump can operate normally and generate a transtubular H$^+$ concentration gradient, resulting in a lowering of the final urine pH. When this occurs, bicarbonate loss ceases and ammonium excretion rises so that a new steady state arises in which acid retention stabilizes, albeit at a reduced plasma bicarbonate concentration.

There are also differences in some of the associated features of proximal *versus* distal RTA. The proximal type may be associated with loss of other molecules normally reabsorbed in the proximal tubule, giving rise to amino aciduria, glycosuria and phosphaturia. A different problem occurs in distal RTA as a result of progressive accumulation of acid over many years. As a consequence of buffering of H$^+$ in bone, calcium is released from the skeleton and may be deposited in the tissues, including the kidney (nephrocalcinosis). Furthermore, the high urinary excretion of calcium may result in stone formation (see Chapter 12), often associated with urinary tract infection. Impairment of skeletal growth can occur in this condition, and also in proximal RTA when the disorder is congenital or starts in early childhood.

Box 4.1 Some causes of renal tubular acidosis (RTA)

Proximal RTA

Congenital (Fanconi syndrome, cystinosis, Wilson's disease)
Paraproteinaemia (e.g. myeloma)
Drugs (carbonic anhydrase inhibitors)

Distal RTA ('classic' type)

Congenital
Hyperglobulinaemia
Autoimmune connective tissue diseases (e.g. systemic lupus erythematosus)
Toxins and drugs (toluene, lithium, amphotericin)

Hyperkalaemic distal RTA

Hypoaldosteronism
Obstructive nephropathy
Renal transplant rejection
Drugs (amiloride, spironolactone)

Much of the symptomatology of both kinds of RTA relates to electrolyte depletion. Urinary losses of sodium are abnormally high in both forms, resulting in a degree of hypovolaemia. Both forms are typically also associated with hypokalaemia because of stimulated potassium secretion in the late distal and cortical collecting ducts. This is caused by a high luminal flow of sodium and bicarbonate in proximal RTA, and by electrically-driven potassium secretion to replace faulty H$^+$ secretion in distal RTA.

An important variant of distal RTA is hyperkalaemic distal RTA (sometimes called type 4 RTA). In this case the normal anion gap metabolic acidosis is associated with hyperkalaemia, which points to a different site of defect in the acid-secreting segment of the nephron. As shown in Fig. 4.7, if a disruption occurs in the normal operation of the principal cell type in this tubular segment, sodium reabsorption will be impaired, resulting in a loss of the normal lumen negativity (see Chapter 2). This electrical change impairs the rate of secretion of both potassium and hydrogen ions into the lumen, resulting in systemic acidosis with hyperkalaemia. This lesion has been described in a variety of conditions causing distal tubulointerstitial damage (such as urinary tract obstruction with infection), and also during treatment with drugs interfering with principal cell sodium transport (such as amiloride). A similar defect results from deficiencies in aldosterone secretion or action, including diseases of the adrenal cortex and of the renin secretory mechanism in the kidney.

The management of all forms of RTA is directed in the first instance toward reversing the underlying condition affecting tubular function, if possible. The next principle is that sufficient bicarbonate buffer must be provided to replace that consumed by the acid being accumulated. Provision of some of this bicarbonate as potassium salt will help replete potassium lost in classic forms of the disorder, while in the hyperkalaemic variant of distal RTA, measures to assist in the excretion of potassium (e.g. loop or thiazide diuretics, or corticosteroids, as appropriate) may be necessary. Treatment may also be required for specific complications in the various forms of the condition, such as removal of stones and treatment of infections which sometimes complicate classic distal RTA.

Case 4.1 Acid–base balance and regulation of pH: 4

Treatment and outcome

Mrs Loy's treatment focused on the control of her underlying connective tissue disease. Immunosuppression using prednisone and cyclophosphamide was initiated with a view to reducing the activity of her SLE. The metabolic acidosis and hypokalaemia were corrected initially with infusions, and later with oral supplements, of alkaline salts of sodium and potassium.

Over the ensuing weeks her condition improved dramatically, with the fevers and rash subsiding, urinary protein and red cell excretion reduced, and plasma electrolyte profile reverted towards normal. Within several weeks it was possible to discontinue her electrolyte and buffer therapy, and ongoing management was directed towards long-term stabilization of the connective tissue disease.

Disturbances of acid–base balance: alkalosis

To complete our survey of acid–base disturbances, we can consider the two primary perturbations which might result in alkalosis.

Respiratory alkalosis

Any form of sustained hyperventilation will produce a reduction in the blood pCO_2 with a resulting increase in plasma pH. The respiratory stimulus most commonly arises from anxiety states, but it may also be due to drugs stimulating the respiratory centre, other brain disorders and chronic liver disease.

The homeostatic response to respiratory alkalosis involves an initial phase of physicochemical buffering by intracellular proteins, which give up H^+, resulting in a small decrease in the plasma bicarbonate. More sustained compensation occurs over the ensuing days, during which renal tubular H^+ secretion is inhibited by the high extracellular pH and the reduced pCO_2. Bicarbonate reabsorption is inhibited, as is ammonium excretion, and the result is a reduction in net acid excretion and a fall in the plasma bicarbonate. In many cases the respiratory disturbance is not unduly prolonged, and the renal compensation subsides as ventilation is normalized.

Metabolic alkalosis

In this disorder there is a primary increase in the plasma bicarbonate concentration and the plasma pH. The causes fall into two groups according to whether there is associated contraction of the ECF volume or not.

Hypovolaemic metabolic alkalosis is the commonest pattern, and includes disorders such as vomiting and gastric suction, in which acid-rich gastric juices are lost from the body. Metabolic alkalosis associated with volume contraction also occurs during treatment with most diuretics (other than carbonic anhydrase inhibitors and potassium-sparing drugs). Here there is increased acid loss into the urine related to the diuretic action on the tubules. The alkalosis associated with volume contraction is perpetuated by secondary renal responses, described in more detail below.

Normovolaemic (or hypervolaemic) metabolic alkalosis occurs when the primary disturbance provokes both bicarbonate retention and a degree of volume expansion. This most commonly occurs in corticosteroid excess states such as primary hyperaldosteronism (Conn's syndrome), Cushing's syndrome and related disorders. Potassium loss in these conditions also contributes to the systemic alkalosis as H^+ ions move into cells in exchange for K^+ ions moving into the ECF. Occasionally, overuse of antacid salts can produce a similar pattern though without external potassium imbalance.

The homeostatic response to metabolic alkalosis involves initial buffering of the rise in plasma bicarbonate by titration of extracellular and intracellular buffers, including plasma proteins. Soon afterwards, the increased pH acts to inhibit ventilation through the medullary chemoreceptors, such that the pCO_2 starts to rise. Since, however, this is ultimately associated with an unacceptable degree of hypoxia, the extent to which this form of compensation occurs is limited, such that the maximum pCO_2 attained is rarely more than 55 mm Hg.

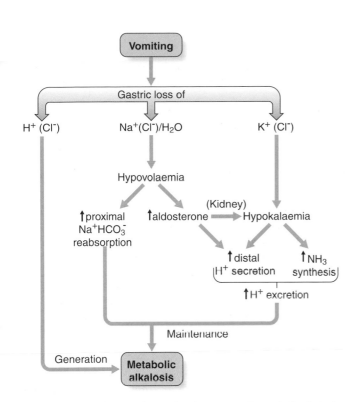

Fig. 4.8 Vomiting: generation and maintenance of metabolic alkalosis. Note that the gastric loss of H$^+$ is primarily responsible for generating the systemic alkalosis, while the other mechanisms shown act through the kidney to maintain the alkalosis as long as sodium and potassium losses are uncorrected. Chloride is the deficient anion accompanying all cations shown.

In the absence of counterbalancing stimuli, the expected renal response to sustained metabolic alkalosis would be to decrease tubular acid secretion, inhibit bicarbonate reabsorption and excrete the excess bicarbonate into the urine. However, in the commonest form of metabolic alkalosis, that caused by sustained vomiting, this response is distorted by other changes associated with the loss of gastric fluid. As shown in Fig. 4.8, the loss of H$^+$ initiates the alkalosis ('generation' phase), which is actually worsened by the losses of sodium, water and potassium ('maintenance' phase). The sodium losses are associated with hypovolaemia, which triggers both proximal bicarbonate reabsorption and aldosterone release, which stimulates distal acid secretion, thereby aggravating the systemic alkalosis. Furthermore, the hypokalaemia resulting from potassium loss (more through the kidney than from gastric fluid) also stimulates distal acid secretion and tubular ammonia synthesis (see earlier), both of which enhance acid excretion and maintain the alkalosis. The net result is an inappropriately acid urine

and a failure of the kidney to effect long-term correction of the systemic pH disturbance.

The cornerstone of management in hypovolaemic metabolic alkalosis states, exemplified by vomiting, is to provide adequate volume replacement as sodium chloride (isotonic saline infusions), which switches off the volume-conserving mechanisms mentioned above and allows the kidney to excrete the excess alkali in the urine. Replacement of potassium helps correct the hypokalaemia and its consequences in the kidney.

The non-hypovolaemic forms of metabolic alkalosis, by way of contrast, are resistant to treatment with sodium chloride, but can usually be managed by cessation of alkali therapy or correction of mineralocorticoid excess. The latter may involve either adrenal gland surgery or blockade of mineralocorticoid effect in the kidney by treatment with spironolactone.

Summary of findings in principal acid–base disturbances

Table 4.3 provides an overview of the changes in pH, bicarbonate concentration and pCO$_2$ in the four major simple acid–base disorders. Taken in conjunction with clinical information, the results of these analyses are usually sufficient to enable a diagnosis to be made of the nature and cause of the disturbance. Rules of thumb are available to indicate the predicted compensatory change in pCO$_2$ or bicarbonate levels expected in each of the simple (uncomplicated) acid–base disorders. When the available data for a given patient are not consistent with these changes, a complex or 'mixed' acid–base disorder can be inferred, and the elements of the disturbance usually deduced in conjunction with a thorough clinical evaluation.

Table 4.3 Summary of 'simple' acid–base disturbances

Disorder	pH	Primary change	Compensatory response
Metabolic acidosis	Decreased	Decreased HCO$_3$	Decreased pCO$_2$
Metabolic alkalosis	Increased	Increased HCO$_3$	Increased pCO$_2$
Respiratory acidosis	Decreased	Increased pCO$_2$	Increased HCO$_3$
Respiratory alkalosis	Increased	Decreased pCO$_2$	Decreased HCO$_3$

GLOMERULAR FILTRATION AND ACUTE KIDNEY INJURY

5

Chapter objectives

After studying this chapter you should be able to:

1. Define the determinants of renal blood flow and glomerular filtration.

2. Describe the mechanism of glomerular filtration.

3. Understand the factors that govern autoregulation within the kidney.

4. Understand the concept of clearance and be familiar with the different methods of assessment of renal function.

5. Determine whether oliguria is physiological or due to established renal failure.

6. Recognize the clinical circumstances in which acute kidney injury is likely to occur.

7. Describe the cellular and biochemical mechanisms which underlie acute kidney injury caused by acute tubular necrosis.

8. Outline a logical clinical, laboratory and radiological approach to the assessment of a patient presenting with renal failure.

9. Define the acute clinical complications and the biochemical and haematological abnormalities in acute kidney injury.

10. Effectively anticipate, prevent and treat the complications occurring in acute kidney injury.

Introduction

As described in previous chapters, the primary functions of the kidney are to maintain body fluid, electrolyte and acid–base homeostasis, and to excrete nitrogenous wastes. These functions rely on a normal anatomical outflow pathway, a normal renal circulation, and normal intrarenal mechanisms for regulating the process of urine formation. Abnormalities in any of these structures or processes can underlie the development of acute kidney injury (also called acute renal failure), characterized by an abrupt fall in glomerular filtration rate (GFR). After studying this chapter you should be able to describe the mechanism of glomerular filtration, the factors normally involved in its regulation, and the causes, consequences and treatment of acute kidney injury. See 5.1:1.

Renal blood flow

Renal blood flow is between 1.0 and 1.2 litres per minute per $1.73\,m^2$ of body surface area. The majority of blood flow to the kidney is directed to the cortex, with only a small proportion delivered to the medulla, where sodium transport by the thick ascending limb of the loop of Henle accounts for a high oxygen consumption. Thus the renal medulla is sensitive to reductions in renal blood flow and oxygen delivery that may induce hypoxia and result in tubular damage, causing acute kidney injury.

The main determinant of the overall renal blood flow is the state of vasoconstriction of the renal arterial tree. Changes in the intrarenal vascular resistance mediate significant alterations in renal blood flow under pathophysiological conditions, while over a wide range of physiological mean arterial pressure levels, renal vasoregulation contributes to the maintenance of a stable renal blood flow and hence GFR (see below, under Autoregulation).

Glomerular filtration

As described earlier in this book, the key process involved in the kidney's excretory function is the formation of an ultrafiltrate of plasma in the glomeruli, where capillary tufts arising from the arterial circulation meet the blind ends of the tubular system in which urine is modified and conducted into the urine drainage system.

The structure of the glomerulus will be discussed in detail in Chapter 6. In brief, the process of filtration occurs across a complex barrier consisting of the thin **fenestrated** endothelial lining of the glomerular capillary, the glomerular basement membrane, and the foot processes of the epithelial cells (derived from the end of the tubular system) apposed to the external wall of the capillary. This filtration barrier allows free passage of solutes (up to a molecular weight of around 60,000 D), but retains cells and protein within the circulation. The selective properties of this barrier, and the consequences of its disruption, will be discussed further in the next two chapters.

The filtration process itself is based on purely passive forces, of which the hydrostatic pressure generated by the heart is the principal driving force. However, as shown in Fig. 5.1, this outward filtration pressure is partially opposed by two pressures acting to restrain filtration, namely the hydrostatic pressure within the lumen of the tubular system itself, and by the oncotic pressure due to plasma proteins which are retained within the capillary. Thus the net ultrafiltration pressure (P_{uf}) comprises the hydrostatic pressure in the glomerular capillaries (P_{gc}) minus the hydrostatic pressure in the tubules (P_t) minus the oncotic pressure generated by plasma proteins (π_{gc}).

An overall expression for GFR which indicates all of its determinants is as follows:

$$GFR = K_f \times P_{uf}$$

where K_f is the ultrafiltration coefficient, which is made up of the product of the hydraulic permeability of the filtration membrane times the surface area available for filtration.

Typical mean values for the pressure terms (obtained from micropuncture studies in experimental animals) indicate that: $P_{gc} = 45\,mm\,Hg$, $P_t = 10\,mm\,Hg$, ($\pi_{gc} = 25\,mm\,Hg$, giving rise to a net ultrafiltration pressure P_{uf} of $10\,mm\,Hg$.

Factors which interfere with any of these determinants of glomerular filtration may lead to an abrupt fall in GFR and thus acute kidney injury unless adequate compensatory responses occur. The most important physiological determinant is the capillary hydrostatic pressure, which may be reduced either by a reduction in perfusion pressure reaching the afferent arteriole, by an increase in afferent arteriolar tone, or by a decrease in efferent arteriolar tone (see below). The pressure in the tubular system may rise significantly during ureteric obstruction, thus reducing the GFR. Changes in the plasma oncotic pressure are less important in altering GFR under physiological or pathological conditions. Pathological change involving the glomeruli may lead to alterations in the ultrafiltration coefficient by decreasing the hydraulic permeability and/or by obliterating the total capillary surface area available for filtration. Conditions such as glomerulonephritis (see Chapter 7) and diabetes mellitus (see Chapter 8) impair glomerular filtration by these mechanisms.

Under physiological conditions, the regulation of the filtration rate in individual glomeruli is determined by the balance between the resistance in the afferent and efferent arterioles. As shown in Fig. 5.2, the hydrostatic pressure across the wall of the glomerular capillaries will be increased by factors either dilating the afferent arteriole, or constricting the efferent arteriole, increasing the single nephron GFR in either case. Conversely, factors leading to afferent arteriolar constriction or efferent

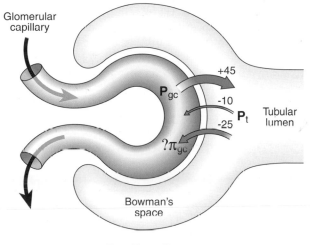

$$P_{uf} = P_{gc} - P_t - \pi_{gc}$$

Fig. 5.1 Diagram of glomerulus showing the forces involved in glomerular filtration. P_{uf}, net ultrafiltration pressure; P_{gc}, hydrostatic pressure in glomerular capillary; P_t, hydrostatic pressure in tubular lumen; π_{gc}, oncotic pressure (osmotic pressure due to plasma proteins) in the glomerular capillary. Representative pressures are shown in mm Hg.

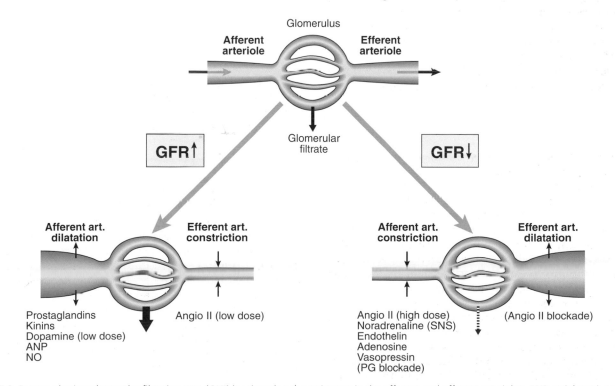

Fig. 5.2 Factors altering glomerular filtration rate (GFR) by changing the resistance in the afferent and efferent arterioles. ANP, atrial natriuretic peptide; Angio II, angiotensin II; NO, nitric oxide; PG, prostaglandin; SNS, sympathetic nervous system.

arteriolar dilatation will reduce the filtration rate of the affected glomerulus. Some circulating substances known to have these effects are shown in Fig. 5.2. It should be noted, however, that in the normal kidney minor perturbations in levels of individual substances do not have significant net effects on GFR because of compensatory changes in other factors which tend to maintain a haemodynamic steady state. However, if renal function is impaired, particularly because of a low renal perfusion pressure (e.g. renal artery stenosis or cardiac failure), maintenance of GFR is highly dependent on intrinsic compensatory mechanisms such as afferent arteriolar vasodilatation (predominantly due to prostaglandins) and efferent arteriolar vasoconstriction (predominantly due to angiotensin II). Thus, factors which interfere with these compensatory mechanisms, such as non-steroidal anti-inflammatory drugs (which inhibit prostaglandin synthesis) and angiotensin-converting enzyme inhibitors or angiotensin II receptor blockers (which interfere with angiotensin II action), blunt these compensatory responses and may precipitate acute kidney injury (see Chapter 14).

It should be noted that angiotensin II has a particularly important but complex role in the regulation of glomerular filtration. While local production of this peptide acts predominantly on the efferent arteriole to maintain single nephron GFR, higher circulating levels are capable of producing afferent arteriolar vasoconstriction which tends to reduce glomerular filtration. Furthermore, angiotensin II causes contraction of the mesangial cells which support the glomerular capillary network, leading to a reduction in surface area available for filtration and so further acting to reduce filtration. The net effect in a particular physiological or pathophysiological circumstance depends on the balance between these actions, as well as other haemodynamic compensations which occur.

Autoregulation of renal blood flow and glomerular filtration rate

Renal blood flow is generally kept constant over a wide range of blood pressures. This phenomenon, called autoregulation, ensures constancy of glomerular filtration and thus solute excretion despite changes in systemic haemodynamics within certain limits (Fig. 5.3). While a variety of neural and vasoactive pathways may be involved in stabilizing the renal blood flow under these conditions, two particular mechanisms have been invoked to explain the autoregulation of GFR.

First, the *myogenic mechanism* refers to the intrinsic capacity of afferent arteriolar smooth muscle cells to increase their state of contraction in response to an increase in renal perfusion pressure. This response, probably mediated by vasoactive agents produced by endothelial cells acting on smooth muscle cells in the afferent arteriole, serves to blunt the transmission of changed arteriolar pressure into the glomerular capillary bed.

The second mechanism is *tubuloglomerular feedback* (TGF). This describes the process whereby the GFR in individual nephrons is regulated according to the rate of solute flow through that nephron. As described in Chapter 2, the juxtaglomerular apparatus consists of a structure at which the distal tubule of a given nephron comes into close proximity with the afferent and efferent arterioles of the same nephron, where the tubular wall becomes specialized as the macula densa (Fig. 5.4; see also Fig. 2.10). Hence, the ionic composition (and indirectly, the flow rate) of the tubular fluid can be sensed by the macula densa, which signals directly to the vascular

Fig. 5.3 Autoregulation of renal blood flow (RBF) and glomerular filtration rate (GFR).

Fig. 5.4 Tubuloglomerular feedback. [NaCl] refers to the concentration of NaCl in the luminal fluid at the macula densa (top of the ascending limb of the loop of Henle). The inset shows the shape of the relationship between the [NaCl] at the macula densa and the glomerular filtration rate (GFR) in the same nephron.

structures of the glomerulus to influence GFR. In brief, during conditions of avid tubular sodium chloride reabsorption, the sodium chloride concentration of the luminal fluid is reduced at the macula densa. Filtration in the corresponding glomerulus is increased, primarily by dilatation of the afferent arteriole. Conversely, when sodium chloride concentration and fluid delivery are high at the macula densa, afferent arteriolar tone is increased and single nephron GFR falls. This feedback mechanism, probably designed to limit the loss of fluid and electrolytes from damaged nephrons, also contributes to the process of autoregulation. This is because increases in renal perfusion pressure would, of themselves, tend to lead to increased filtration and solute loss, which TGF effectively blunts. The mediator of the vasoconstrictor response involved in TGF appears to be locally produced adenosine, acting via the adenosine 1 receptor on the afferent arteriole. It is possible that other vasoactive mechanisms also play a part.

Renal excretion and the clearance formula

The rate at which a solute (s) is excreted by the kidney (E_s) is given simply by the product of the concentration of the solute in the urine (U_s) and the urine flow rate (V), which is the urine volume over a defined period. That is:

$$E_s = U_s \times V$$

where the units of E are mmol/min (or equivalent). This expression is useful in assessing absolute removal rates of solute by the kidney, and hence evaluating total body mass balance.

The renal clearance (C_s) of solute (s) on the other hand, is defined as the apparent volume of plasma from which the substance is completely removed per unit time during passage through the kidneys. It is equivalent mathematically to the ratio of the excretion rate to the simultaneous plasma concentration for that substance (P_s):

$$C_s = (U_s \times V)/P_s$$

The units of clearance are mL/min (or equivalent). The clearance calculation provides a measure of the relative efficiency of the kidney in removing a given solute from the plasma, and a means of comparison between substances which are handled differently by the nephron. The range of possible clearance rates is from zero (for a substance which is either not filtered at all or is filtered and then completely reabsorbed by the tubular system) up to a maximum equivalent to the renal plasma flow rate (for a substance which is filtered and totally secreted by the tubular system). Interpretation of clearance calculations depends on knowing whether the substance is freely filtered at the glomerulus. The procedure requires the presence of a steady state in the plasma concentration throughout the time frame of the period under study.

Measuring the glomerular filtration rate

The utility of the clearance concept in renal physiology is illustrated best by its application to the determination of GFR. As shown in Fig. 5.5, the renal handling of the plant polysaccharide inulin is such that it is freely filtered at the glomerulus and undergoes no reabsorption or secretion during its passage through the tubular system. It follows from simple mass balance that the amount being filtered into the early part of the tubular system equals the amount being excreted at the end of that system. As shown in Fig. 5.5, this gives rise to the inference that the GFR can be measured by determining the clearance of inulin, which is possible experimentally simply by measuring its concentration in the

Fig. 5.5 Schematic illustration of the application of the clearance concept to the determination of the glomerular filtration rate (GFR). P_{in}, inulin concentration in plasma brought to the glomerulus; U_{in}, inulin concentration in final urine; V, urine flow rate; C_{in}, clearance of inulin.

plasma and urine, as well as the urine flow rate, during a steady state infusion.

Unfortunately, there are logistical difficulties involved in determining inulin clearance since it needs to be infused and is difficult to assay. While a variety of other substances behave in a way similar to inulin and can be used clinically (e.g. iothalamate), in practice a great advantage is gained by using the clearance of an endogenous molecule whose behaviour approximates that of inulin for clinical determination of GFR. Such a substance is creatinine, derived from the metabolic breakdown of creatine, a component of skeletal muscle. For a given individual, the amount of creatinine entering the circulation per day is dependent almost exclusively on the skeletal muscle mass. As long as renal function is stable, this same daily amount will be excreted in the urine, given by the product of U_{cr} and V. Creatinine, like inulin, is freely filtered at the glomerulus and undergoes no tubular reabsorption, although there is a small degree of secretion by the tubules when renal function is impaired. None the less, under most conditions the clearance of endogenous creatinine provides a measure of GFR which is sufficiently robust for clinical use. Moreover, because $U_{cr} \times V$ is a constant (k) for a given individual under steady state conditions, there is a fixed relationship between the GFR and plasma creatinine, in the form of a rectangular hyperbola as shown in Fig. 5.6.

Several important deductions can be made from inspection of this relationship. First, plasma creatinine only starts to increase substantially when approximately 50% of renal function (GFR) is lost. Thus, a significant reduction in GFR can be present before the plasma creatinine is recorded outside the 'normal' reference range for a laboratory. Second, each such relationship is specific to a given individual with a particular muscle mass, making comparison of plasma creatinine between patients of different morphology difficult. For example, in patients with a low muscle mass, particularly elderly females,

plasma creatinine can lie within the normal range in the presence of marked reductions in renal function. This is equivalent to saying that patients with increasing muscle masses have different GFR *versus* plasma creatinine graphs, displaced to the right in Fig. 5.6 for increasing muscle mass.

To obviate some of these difficulties in interpretation of plasma creatinine, a number of nomograms have been devised which give a reasonably accurate estimate of GFR from the plasma creatinine in an individual of a certain age, weight and gender. One such formula is that of Cockcroft and Gault, namely:

$$\text{Estimated GFR (mL/min)} = \frac{(140 - \text{age}) \times \text{weight (kg)}}{814 \times \text{plasma creatinine (mmol/L)}}$$

The result should be multiplied by 0.85 for women to allow for the relatively lower proportion of body weight which is muscle. This formula has proved useful in the modification of drug doses in the context of reduced GFR.

However, the formula most widely used at present to estimate GFR is derived from the Modification of Diet in Renal Disease (MDRD) study. This study derived an equation validated for the measurement of GFR in Caucasian and African-American populations with mild to moderate renal impairment, based on the variables race, gender, age and plasma creatinine (weight is not required). The equation is as follows but a result is automatically generated by several calculators available on the internet.

$$\text{GFR (mL/min/1.73 m}^2) = 32788 \times (P_{cr})^{-1.154} \times (\text{Age})^{-0.203} \times (0.742 \text{ if female}) \times (1.212 \text{ if African-American})$$

The units for plasma creatinine (P_{cr}) in this version of the equation are micromol/L.

It is important to recognize that this formula for estimated GFR (or eGFR) does not take the patient's actual body size into account, but yields an adjusted GFR normalized to an average adult body surface area of 1.73 m². Note also that validation for Asian and indigenous populations has not to date been performed.

Hence at present, it is recommended that the MDRD formula is used to estimate GFR in Caucasian and African-American patients with a GFR between 15 and 60 mL/min. In adjusting drug doses based on renal function, the Cockroft and Gault formula should be used since the MDRD equation has not been validated for this purpose in patients with renal impairment.

Urea

Urea is one of the main metabolic products of protein metabolism, and its excretion into the urine is one of the key functions of the kidney. Urea ($NH_2.CO.NH_2$) is synthesized in the liver from ammonium ions, derived from amino acid catabolism, plus carbon dioxide. It is freely

Fig. 5.6 Relationship between creatinine clearance (an estimate of glomerular filtration rate) and plasma creatinine concentration. C_{cr}, creatinine clearance; U_{cr}, urine creatinine concentration; V, urine flow rate; P_{cr}, plasma creatinine concentration. k_1 represents the curve for a small–average patient, while k_2 and k_3 show the position of the curve for progressively heavier patients.

filtered at the glomerulus, but undergoes approximately 50% reabsorption during passage through the nephron. Thus the clearance of urea is approximately half the GFR, and plasma urea varies inversely with the GFR. However, the fraction of filtered urea which is reabsorbed is not constant, being greater during conditions of dehydration and low urine flow rate. This makes urea less valuable as a direct measure of GFR than creatinine, since it is influenced not only by the GFR but also by the state of hydration. Furthermore, urea production is related to the amount of protein absorbed from the gut and to the protein catabolic rate (Box 5.2). Consideration of the factors in this box allows for an informed interpretation of the results of plasma creatinine and urea levels. This will be of value later in our consideration of Mrs Campbell.

Pathophysiology of oliguria

We turn now to a consideration of the origin and significance of the greatly reduced urine volume in the present patient. The urinary volume varies widely on a daily basis in normal individuals because of regulatory mechanisms aimed at maintaining a normal and constant body fluid volume. As described in Chapter 2, the main factors that are regulated to control body fluid volume and osmolality are the rates of reabsorption of sodium and water during their passage through the nephron. During states of sodium depletion and extracellular fluid (ECF) volume contraction, sodium reabsorptive mechanisms are activated, resulting in excretion of urine with a low sodium content. Similarly, during water deprivation, the kidney can concentrate urine sufficiently to maintain water balance at an intake of less than 500 mL/day. This capacity is largely related to the anatomical and physiological integrity of the tubular structures within the renal

medulla, and their responsiveness to antidiuretic hormone, which is released during states of dehydration.

Thus, a low urine flow rate itself may be a normal response to hypovolaemia, often accompanied by systemic and renal haemodynamic changes ('prerenal' oliguria). By definition, acute kidney injury is only present when there is evidence for a reduced GFR; indeed, this diagnosis can be made in the presence of a normal or even increased urine volume under certain circumstances. However, when there is sustained oliguria, defined as a urine volume of less than 400 mL/24h, the likelihood of a low GFR is increased, but it is necessary to establish whether this is essentially 'physiological' and reversible, or pathological and indicative of structural renal damage.

The clinical history and examination are often helpful in suggesting which of these patterns of oliguria is present in a particular patient. Thus, sustained hypovolaemia or shock, or the presence of toxins known to cause tubular necrosis (see below), suggests that widespread damage to the parenchyma is likely, while shorter lived or lesser insults make 'physiological' oliguria more likely. A number of biochemical measurements have been found to provide assistance in making this differentiation. As shown in Table 5.1, markers of functional oliguria on a prerenal basis are those predicted by the expected physiological responses outlined above: thus urinary sodium concentration and fractional sodium excretion are low in this setting, but high when tubular damage is established. Osmolality and creatinine concentrations are high in the urine in prerenal oliguria, and low when damage is established. As predicted by the above discussion of factors influencing plasma urea and creatinine concentrations, the ratio of plasma urea to creatinine is high in prerenal oliguria, and lower in tubular necrosis.

In broad terms, the functional oliguria associated with physiological responses to hypovolaemia is reversible with appropriate fluid replacement therapy, while that associated with structural damage is less likely to be so. Thus, making this differentiation has important therapeutic implications, as will be illustrated later in the present patient. See Case 5.1 in Box 3.

Box 5.1 Factors causing an increase in plasma creatinine and urea concentrations

Creatinine	Urea
Decreased GFR	Decreased GFR
Increased skeletal muscle mass (long-term)	Decreased urine flow rate
	Increased protein intake:
	Diet
	Gastrointestinal bleeding
	Increased protein catabolic rate:
	Sepsis
	Steroid therapy
	Some tetracycline antibiotics
GFR, glomerular filtration rate.	

Table 5.1 Laboratory assessment to differentiate prerenal oliguria from established renal failure

Laboratory parameter	Prerenal	Established renal failure
Urinary [Na] (mmol/L)	<20	>40
Fractional Na excretion[*]	<1%	>1%
Urine:plasma osmolality ratio	>1.5	<1.1
Urine:plasma creatinine ratio	>40	<20
Plasma urea:creatinine ratio (both in mmol/L)	>80	<80

*Fractional excretion of Na (FE_{Na})

$$= \frac{(Urine_{Na}/Plasma_{Na})}{(Urine_{Cr}/Plasma_{Cr})} \times 100\%$$

Glomerular filtration and acute kidney injury: 2

Investigations

Initial blood tests in Mrs Campbell showed an elevation in the white cell count, with a neutrophilia consistent with infection. The haemoglobin was *168 g/L and haematocrit was *0.53, consistent with haemoconcentration.

The plasma urea concentration was elevated at *26 mmol/L and creatinine was elevated at *0.35 mmol/L. The plasma sodium was 145 mmol/L and the potassium was elevated at *6.1 mmol/L. Acidosis was present, indicated by the reduced bicarbonate at *18 mmol/L. The serum albumin was 48 g/L, calcium was 2.20 mmol/L and phosphate was *1.8 mmol/L.

Biochemical analysis of the urine specimen taken on admission revealed a urinary sodium concentration of 44 mmol/L and a creatinine concentration of 6.5 mmol/L. The urine osmolality was 335 mosm/kg (compare plasma of 302 mosm/kg).

From these data we can conclude that Mrs Campbell's oliguria is in fact associated with acute kidney injury, given the marked elevation of plasma creatinine which implies a reduced GFR. The urine parameters are suggestive of impaired renal tubular function consistent with acute tubular necrosis (ATN).

The questions now arise:

1. What has caused the acute kidney injury in this case?
2. What is the pathology and natural history of ATN?
3. How have the plasma biochemistry abnormalities come about?
4. What complications of acute kidney injury can be anticipated and treated?

*Results outside the normal range; see Appendix.

Causes of acute kidney injury

Acute kidney injury (also called acute renal failure) is a clinical term that encompasses many causes of abrupt renal impairment; that is, a fall in GFR occurring over a period of hours or days which results in impaired fluid and electrolyte homeostasis and the accumulation of nitrogenous wastes. Acute kidney injury occurs in response to a wide variety of insults, the most common causes being haemodynamic, immunological, toxic and obstructive. Classically, the causes of acute kidney injury are divided into prerenal, renal and postrenal causes depending on the site of the initiating insult (Table 5.2).

The commonest causes of acute kidney injury acquired out of hospital are prolonged ischaemic injury in some 50% of cases, and nephrotoxic injury in 35%. In hospital-acquired renal failure, the cause is usually multifactorial. The major predisposing factors include volume depletion (often caused by vomiting, diarrhoea or diuretics), and treatment with drugs (such as angiotensin-converting enzyme inhibitors, angiotensin II receptor blockers or non-steroidal anti-inflammatory drugs), and radiocontrast

Table 5.2 Causes of acute kidney injury

Prerenal	Renal	Postrenal
Hypovolaemia	Acute tubular necrosis (ischaemic or toxic)	Bilateral ureteric obstruction
Decreased effective blood volume	Interstitial nephritis (e.g. drugs – see Chapter 14)	Ureteric obstruction in a single kidney
Decreased cardiac output	Glomerular disease (e.g. acute glomerulonephritis)	Bladder outflow obstruction
Renovascular obstruction	Small vessel disease (e.g. microvasculitis)	
	Intrarenal vasoconstriction (e.g. in sepsis)	
	Tubular obstruction (e.g. urate crystals)	

agents. Elderly, diabetic and chronically hypertensive patients are at particular risk because of their predisposition to underlying vascular disease and poor renal autoregulatory responses. In the hospital population, hypotension, heart failure, sepsis and aminoglycoside use are common additional factors involved in the genesis of acute kidney injury. Sustained circulatory impairment leading to ischaemia-induced ATN accounts for the majority of cases of acute kidney injury overall.

Acute tubular necrosis

When the kidney sustains a severe hypoxic insult, injury and death of tubular cells occurs, and the resulting clinicopathological syndrome is referred to as ATN. This most commonly occurs as a result of prolonged renal ischaemia during a period of hypotension. Other causes include direct toxic injury to the tubules by endogenous chemicals such as myoglobin (released from damaged muscle cells – rhabdomyolysis) or haemoglobin (released from red blood cells during acute episodes of haemolysis). Less commonly, ATN results from exposure to nephrotoxic drugs (see Chapter 11) and heavy metals.

A number of biochemical processes have been implicated in the development of injury to tubular cells, particularly following the onset of renal ischaemia. These include depletion of cellular ATP, increase in intracellular calcium, disruption of cytoskeletal structures, loss of epithelial polarity, activation of apoptosis (programmed cell death), and increased oxygen free radical production. The latter mechanism may be particularly important as a cause of tissue injury during the reperfusion phase after a period of ischaemia.

Pathology of acute tubular necrosis

Histologically, the changes in ATN are most prominent in the cells of the proximal tubule, particularly in its latter

Fig. 5.7 Micrograph (stained with haematoxylin and eosin) showing acute tubular necrosis. Note the atrophy of the tubular epithelium, the dilatation of tubules and the interstitial oedema (wide separation between adjacent tubules).

third (S3 segment). Blebs appear in the apical brush border, with sloughing of the brush border membrane into the lumen or involution into the cytoplasm. The integrity of the tight junctions is disrupted and loss of epithelial cell polarity occurs. Integrins, which normally contribute to cell–cell adhesion, are redistributed to the apical membrane, resulting in shedding of both live and dead cells into the lumen, which contributes to cast formation and tubular obstruction. Interstitial oedema is prominent because of leakage of tubular fluid across damaged tubular walls (Fig. 5.7). The glomeruli are generally relatively well preserved.

Pathophysiology of acute tubular necrosis

A variety of mechanisms have been proposed to explain the persistence of reduced glomerular filtration in the context of ATN, even after the instigating stimulus has been corrected or removed. These include sustained renal vasoconstriction, probably mediated by intrarenal humoral factors, reduced glomerular permeability, mechanical obstruction by sloughed cells and proteinaceous casts, and back-leak of filtrate from the tubular lumen. It is likely that a different pattern of mechanisms is involved depending on the exact cause or contributing factors in a given case of ATN.

Course of acute tubular necrosis

Impaired renal function and oligoanuria during ATN typically persist for 1 week or more, after which complete cellular recovery can occur, accompanied by a return of GFR towards normal and a marked increase in urine output. This recovery is due to epithelial cell regeneration, probably under the control of locally produced peptide growth factors such as insulin-like growth factor 1 and epidermal growth factor.

Case 5.1 Glomerular filtration and acute kidney injury: 3

Progress

Mrs Campbell's acute kidney injury was attributed to ATN on the basis of prolonged renal ischaemia caused by dehydration, hypotension and sepsis, on a background of treatment with a diuretic and an angiotensin-converting enzyme (ACE) inhibitor.

Initial treatment consisted of ceasing her antihypertensives, rehydration with normal saline and commencement of intravenous antibiotics (ampicillin 1g tds, metronidazole 500mg tds and gentamicin 240mg in a single initial dose). A surgical opinion was sought, and a conservative approach to management of her diverticular abscess was recommended in the first instance.

Over the following 2 days, Mrs Campbell's general condition improved considerably, with loss of fever and improvement of tissue hydration, with the blood pressure rising to 150/85. However, her urine output remained very poor and the plasma creatinine concentration increased further to *0.45mmol/L. Mild hyperkalaemia and acidosis persisted.

In view of these developments, consistent with a sustained reduction in GFR due to tubular necrosis, Mrs Campbell was seen by the consultant nephrologist who arranged for her to commence intermittent haemodialysis via a temporary catheter inserted into her jugular vein. She tolerated these treatments well, and there was further improvement in her clinical condition and electrolytes over the following week. She received parenteral nutrition over this period.

Ten days after admission, an increase in urine output was noted, which was then matched by an increase in her intravenous fluid therapy. Over the next few days, her plasma urea and creatinine concentrations started to fall towards normal, and her dialysis was discontinued. She was now eating and drinking, and was recommenced on an antihypertensive drug regime to control her blood pressure. On surgical review, the decision was made to defer surgery on her bowel until further settling of her inflammatory mass had occurred. She was discharged from hospital 2 weeks after admission.

As long as renal function can be temporarily replaced with a form of dialysis during the period of suppressed GFR, with correction of electrolyte disturbances and maintenance of adequate nutrition the patient can recover and reattain normal renal function. Close attention to replacement of fluid and electrolytes is important during the early recovery phase, as a period of polyuria and uncontrolled electrolyte loss is common as tubular regeneration proceeds. See 5.1:3.

Overview: assessment and management of a patient with acute kidney injury

A logical approach to the evaluation of a patient with acute kidney injury is presented in Table 5.3. All patients

Table 5.3 Assessment of a patient with acute kidney injury

Procedure	Information sought
Clinical history and examination	Clues to the cause of acute kidney injury (see Table 5.2)
	Indicators of severity of metabolic disturbance
	Estimate of volume status (hydration) (see Table 2.1)
Urinalysis and urine microscopy	Markers of glomerular or tubulointerstitial inflammation, urinary tract infection or crystal uropathy
Plasma biochemistry	To assess extent of GFR reduction and metabolic consequences
Urine biochemistry	To differentiate prerenal from established renal failure (see Table 5.1)
Full blood count	To determine presence of anaemia, leucocytosis and platelet consumption
Renal ultrasound	To determine kidney size, presence of obstruction, abnormal renal parenchymal texture
Plus, where appropriate:	
Abdominal CT scan*	To define structural abnormalities of the kidneys or urinary tract
Radionuclide scan	To assess abnormal renal perfusion
Cystoscopy±retrograde pyelograms	To evaluate/relieve urinary tract obstruction
Renal biopsy	To define pathology of renal parenchymal disease

*CT, computed tomography; note that this should generally be performed without the use of contrast agent in the context of impaired GFR.

presenting with acute kidney injury require a careful history and examination, urinalysis and urine microscopy, plasma and urine biochemistry analysis and full blood count. In general, urinary tract obstruction should be excluded early on with a renal ultrasound. Subsequent investigations depend on whether the cause of acute kidney injury is considered to be caused by prerenal, renal or postrenal pathology. Clues should also be sought to determine whether there is a background of chronic kidney disease, which is suggested by anaemia, hyperphosphataemia, hypocalcaemia and small kidney size.

Biochemical changes in acute kidney injury

When the kidneys fail over a short time period, the metabolic disturbances which occur reflect failure of their normal homeostatic role in maintaining body fluid volume and composition within a narrow normal range. Changes in plasma biochemistry usually seen in this situation are shown in Box 5.2. It is important to note that

Box 5.2 Changes in plasma biochemistry in acute kidney injury

> Hyperkalaemia
> Decreased bicarbonate
> Elevated urea
> Elevated creatinine
> Elevated uric acid
> Hypocalcaemia
> Hyperphosphataemia

this box does not include any direct indication of altered body fluid volume in acute kidney injury. As a result of an impaired capacity to excrete fluid, this is usually manifested as hypervolaemia and, in extreme cases, pulmonary oedema, which must be assessed clinically and radiologically.

Hyperkalaemia results in part from potassium retention due to a failure of filtration and tubular secretion of potassium by the damaged kidney. There is, in addition, an increased endogenous potassium load associated with some causes of acute kidney injury such as muscle crush injury. This electrolyte disturbance is particularly serious because of its potential to produce life-threatening cardiac asystole through its effect on the excitability of cardiac conducting tissue. It can also lead to profound skeletal muscle weakness.

Other factors which may contribute to hyperkalaemia include conditions or drugs which directly influence the capacity of the distal tubule to secrete potassium, as is sometimes seen in cases where the urinary tract is infected and obstructed, or in low aldosterone states, or when potassium-sparing diuretics or ACE inhibitors are being used. Metabolic acidosis, itself a consequence of acute kidney injury and associated conditions, also frequently contributes to hyperkalaemia by promoting transcellular exchange of potassium ions for hydrogen ions.

ECG abnormalities are often the first indication that severe hyperkalaemia is present (Fig. 5.8). Such changes, usually associated with a serum potassium greater than 6.5 mmol/L, require emergency treatment with an infusion of calcium gluconate to stabilize the membrane potential in the cardiac conducting tissue, followed by agents to shift potassium into cells (nebulized beta-agonists, intravenous sodium bicarbonate, intravenous glucose and insulin). These measures must be accompanied by interventions to remove potassium from the body (ion exchange resins or dialysis).

Metabolic acidosis (reflected by a low bicarbonate) occurs in renal failure because of the retention of organic acids, and failure of the kidney to secrete and excrete the net hydrogen ion load (see Chapter 4). An additional acid load may be generated in some settings of acute kidney injury, such as with lactate production in the presence of poor tissue perfusion.

Elevated urea and creatinine are manifestations of the retention of nitrogenous products of metabolism because

Fig. 5.8 Electrocardiogram in severe hyperkalaemia. Note the widening of the QRS complex and the high peaked T waves compared to the normal tracing. The plasma potassium in this patient was 7.6 mmol/L.

of reduced filtration. Both substances have additional significance as markers of the GFR, with creatinine being more useful for this purpose (see above). Clinical manifestations probably relate most to the elevation in urea, which produces the syndrome of uraemia characterized by impaired mental function (drowsiness and confusion), **anorexia,** nausea and vomiting and, in severe cases, **asterixis** and **pericarditis**.

Hyperphosphataemia also results from failure of filtration, but is aggravated in situations in which a high phosphate load is generated (such as tissue breakdown in rhabdomyolysis or **tumour lysis syndrome**). The total plasma calcium is generally low at the onset of acute kidney injury, although this often normalizes or overcorrects as recovery proceeds.

Complications of acute kidney injury

Complications may arise as a result of the renal failure itself or the illnesses associated with the development of renal failure.

The most important factors in contributing to morbidity and mortality rates are cardiovascular complications arising from fluid overload, arrhythmias, acute myocardial ischaemia and hypertension. Systemic infection is another major cause of adverse outcomes in acute kidney injury. This is probably due to the effect of the abnormal metabolic environment on immunological functions, although it often relates directly to the cause of the acute kidney injury, such as Gram-negative septicaemia or burns.

Neurological disturbances often parallel the rate of rise of blood urea, sometimes resulting in a depressed level of consciousness or seizures.

Gastrointestinal haemorrhage occurs frequently in these patients, often on the basis of an impaired coagulation mechanism. This may be caused by a platelet function defect induced by uraemia, reduced tissue integrity

predisposing to bleeding, and sometimes systemic coagulopathy related to the primary cause of renal failure.

Another factor contributing to high morbidity and mortality rates in acute kidney injury is impaired nutritional status. Factors contributing to this may include:

- anorexia in the period before development of renal failure
- a catabolic state commonly associated with renal failure
- uncontrolled acidosis which accelerates protein breakdown
- inadequate provision of nutrients in the early phase of management.

Management of acute kidney injury

The principles of management of acute kidney injury can be summarized as shown in Table 5.4. Note that the table does not include the measures required to correct the underlying cause of acute kidney injury, e.g. relieving urinary tract obstruction when present.

It should be clear from the above that the availability of renal replacement therapy in the form of acute dialysis is of critical importance in saving lives from this medical emergency. This can be a particularly cost-effective form of intervention given that the kidney has the capacity for complete recovery in many of the conditions underlying this presentation.

Table 5.4 Principles of management of acute kidney injury

Problem	*Management*
Fluid volume disturbance	Rehydrate if hypovolaemic; withhold fluid and give high dose diuretic if hypervolaemic; dialysis for resistant pulmonary oedema
Metabolic disturbances:	
Hyperkalaemia	Intravenous calcium, bicarbonate, glucose plus insulin; oral/rectal ion exchange resin; dialysis
Acidosis	Bicarbonate supplements; dialysis
Uraemic syndrome	Dialysis
Infection	Antibiotics ± surgery if appropriate
Bleeding	dDAVP to improve platelet dysfunction; dialysis
Nutritional deficiencies	Enteral or parenteral feeding in conjunction with dialysis

dDAVP, des-amino D-arginine vasopressin, a synthetic analogue of vasopressin (the naturally occurring antidiuretic hormone) which also has the property of enhancing platelet function.

PROTEINURIA AND THE NEPHROTIC SYNDROME

6

Chapter objectives

After studying this chapter you should be able to:

1. Describe the anatomy of the normal glomerulus, including its three cell types and their arrangement, and the structure of the glomerular capillary wall and glomerular basement membrane (GBM).

2. Discuss the components of normal and abnormal proteinuria, and differentiate tubular and glomerular proteinuria.

3. Understand the role of the glomerulus and its components (cells and GBM) in preventing proteinuria.

4. Discuss the pathophysiology and differential diagnosis of oedema.

5. Understand the features and pathophysiology of nephrotic syndrome and its complications.

6. List the main diseases that cause nephrotic syndrome in children and adults.

7. Describe the renal histopathological features of minimal change disease.

8. Discuss the natural history of minimal change disease, and the other major causes of nephrotic syndrome.

9. Discuss the response to treatment of the major causes of nephrotic syndrome.

Introduction

To produce an ultrafiltrate of plasma as the first stage in urine production, the glomerulus must retain plasma proteins within the lumen of its capillary network. This ability to retain plasma proteins by preventing their filtration into the tubular lumen is determined by the size- and charge-selective properties of the glomerular capillary wall (GCW). When diseases damage the integrity of this wall, plasma proteins may escape across it into the tubular lumen.

The proximal segments of the nephron have the capacity to reabsorb and metabolize very efficiently any proteins that appear in the tubular lumen. Under normal circumstances, small plasma proteins which are able to pass across the GCW are taken up (endocytosed) by proximal tubular cells via luminal membrane receptors such as megalin-cubulin on their brush-border membrane, to be broken down in lysosomes. However, protein may appear in the final urine (proteinuria) if the amount filtered by the glomerulus overwhelms tubular reabsorptive mechanisms, or if tubular cells are damaged.

Severe proteinuria may damage the kidney, or have systemic consequences because of loss of albumin and other proteins from the blood.

In this chapter, the causes and consequences of proteinuria will be considered and illustrated by a case of severe proteinuria occurring in a child (see 6.1: 1).

Pathophysiology of oedema formation

Oedema literally means 'swelling', and refers to the accumulation of fluid within the tissues. This fluid is located outside the vascular system in the interstitial space (see Chapter 2).

Under normal circumstances, the balance between hydrostatic and osmotic pressure gradients (Starling's forces) across capillary walls prevents oedema formation (Fig. 6.1A). The hydrostatic pressure of the column of blood within systemic capillaries is determined by the pumping action of the heart and resistance to flow within the arterial tree, and capacitance of the venous system. Capillary hydrostatic pressure varies in different tissues, but is on average about 25 mm Hg. This favours the movement of plasma filtrate into the surrounding interstitial compartment, which has a lower hydrostatic pressure. This hydrostatic pressure gradient is opposed by osmotic forces which favour the movement of fluid from the interstitium (which has a colloid osmotic pressure, or oncotic pressure, of about 1 mm Hg) into the capillary lumen (where plasma proteins exert an oncotic pressure of about 25 mm Hg). In fact, capillary hydrostatic pressure falls along the length of the capillary, whereas capillary oncotic pressure rises as water moves into the interstitial space. Thus these forces favour net water movement into the interstitium at the arterial end of the capillary (hydrostatic > oncotic pressure), balanced under normal

Proteinuria and the nephrotic syndrome: 1

Generalized oedema

Kylie Major presented to her general practitioner (GP) with facial swelling of 3 days duration. Kylie was a 6-year-old girl who had been completely healthy in the past and had had no antecedent illnesses before presentation. Her GP found obvious pitting oedema (swelling which can be indented by digital compression) in her face and around her ankles. Her blood pressure was 95/60. Her jugular venous pressure was normal, her chest was clear to **auscultation** and there was no shifting dullness on percussion of her abdomen, indicating that there was no clinically obvious ascites (free peritoneal fluid). Dipstick analysis of a fresh urine sample was strongly positive for protein but negative for blood. Her GP thought her generalized oedema was most likely caused by proteinuria.

Consideration of the presenting features of this patient leads to the following questions:

1. What are the forces which prevent the development of oedema normally?
2. What are the major diseases that cause oedema? How are the forces opposing oedema formation disrupted in these conditions?
3. How does proteinuria cause oedema?

These questions will be addressed in the first section of this chapter.

conditions by an equivalent movement of water in the other direction at the venous end (oncotic > hydrostatic pressure). Oedema fluid within the interstitial space is limited also by drainage via lymphatic vessels.

The above principles apply to other capillary beds, but the details of the forces involved vary (see, for example, Chapter 5 for a discussion of forces in the glomerulus, a capillary bed designed to achieve net movement of fluid out of the lumen).

Oedema arises because of a localized or generalized disruption of Starling's forces within capillaries, or because of a failure of lymphatic drainage of the interstitial space (Fig. 6.1B). Thus, factors which favour oedema formation include a loss of integrity of the capillary wall, an increase in hydrostatic pressure within the capillary lumen (e.g. caused by high venous pressures within the systemic or pulmonary circulation as occurs in congestive cardiac failure, and within portal veins in **cirrhosis**), reduction in plasma oncotic pressure due to hypoalbuminaemia, or obstruction of lymphatic flow. The main causes of oedema are listed in Table 6.1.

If oedema formation were determined only by Starling's forces in capillaries, then body weight should not increase. However, in most conditions causing generalized oedema

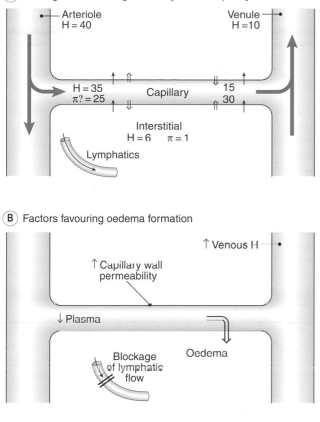

(A) Starling's forces acting across systemic capillary walls

Arteriole
H = 40

Venule
H = 10

H = 35
π? = 25   Capillary   15
30

Interstitial
H = 6   π = 1

Lymphatics

(B) Factors favouring oedema formation

↑ Venous H

↑ Capillary wall
permeability

↓ Plasma

Blockage
of lymphatic
flow

Oedema

H = Hydrostatic   π = Oncotic   → Blood flow   ⇒ Net
pressure   pressure   → Direction   movement
in mm Hg   in mm Hg   of force   of fluid

Fig. 6.1 (A) Starling's forces acting across systemic capillary walls. The net movement of fluid depends on the balance between capillary and interstitial hydrostatic (H) and oncotic (π) pressures. Representative values (in mm Hg) are shown. (B) Factors favouring oedema formation. Reduction in plasma oncotic pressure, increase in capillary wall permeability or venous hydrostatic pressure, or lymphatic blockage will increase oedema formation.

(Table 6.1), the kidneys actively retain salt and water, causing weight gain and aggravating the build-up of oedema fluid. Salt and water retention in these circumstances may arise as a response to a reduction in 'effective' arterial blood volume due to impaired cardiac output or loss of fluid from the circulation into the tissues, leading to a number of responses designed to protect against hypovolaemia (see Chapter 2). These responses include systemic haemodynamic changes which occur quickly, and intrarenal changes which lead to salt and water retention over days to weeks. The intrarenal factors include:

- reflex activation of the sympathetic nervous system
- activation of the renin–angiotensin–aldosterone system and vasopressin release
- resistance to the action of natriuretic peptides
- altered glomerular haemodynamics
- peritubular forces in the proximal tubule.

These neuronal, hormonal and intrarenal mechanisms, which together augment sodium reabsorption at multiple sites along the nephron, are discussed in more detail in Chapter 2. It is important to recognize that evidence also exists to suggest that renal salt and water retention may actually precede the development of circulatory changes in these conditions. In the case of the nephrotic syndrome, this may arise as a result of a fall in GFR as glomerular damage progresses, or from unknown mechanisms promoting distal tubular sodium reabsorption early in the course of the disease process.

The predominant site of oedema can give a clue to the aetiology. Thus, with right-sided heart failure, peripheral oedema (affecting the extremities) should be accompanied by a raised jugular venous pressure and hepatic congestion. With left-sided heart failure, pulmonary congestion alone is expected. With cirrhosis, ascites (fluid accumulation in the peritoneal cavity) is seen earlier than in other causes of generalized oedema because of portal venous hypertension. Peripheral oedema also occurs with cirrhosis owing to hypoalbuminaemia.

When there is marked proteinuria, peripheral and/or facial oedema develops because of hypoalbuminaemia. This combination of findings is called the nephrotic syndrome (or nephrosis), which will be discussed further below. The site of oedema is also influenced by the effect of gravity. Thus, in ambulant patients, mild oedema is frequently seen first around the ankles (where venous hydrostatic pressure is highest in the erect posture), whereas in bedridden patients it may be over the sacrum as this is the most dependent position. With severe nephrotic syndrome, oedema can be more widespread and may involve the lungs and pleural and peritoneal cavities. If renal salt and water retention is a predominant pathophysiological event, as occurs in some forms of nephrosis (particularly where the glomerular filtration rate (GFR) is reduced), the blood volume may be increased and jugular venous pressure raised.

The three main generalized oedema states are congestive cardiac failure, cirrhosis and nephrotic syndrome. These may be differentiated by the finding of signs of cardiac disease in the case of congestive cardiac failure, of liver failure in the case of cirrhosis, and of heavy proteinuria in cases of nephrotic syndrome. The latter is clearly the problem in the present patient and will be the subject of the rest of this chapter.

Glomerular anatomy and the filtration barrier

Each human kidney contains about one million glomeruli, each of which is a specialized capillary network fed by a single afferent arteriole and drained by a single efferent arteriole. The glomerulus is populated by three intrinsic cells: the capillary endothelial cell, the epithelial cell which lies over it with the glomerular basement membrane (GBM) in between, and the mesangial cell.

Table 6.1 Main causes of oedema

	Pathophysiological factors	Predominant site
Local		
Infection, trauma	Capillary leak	Local
Venous obstruction (e.g. thrombosis)	Increased venous hydrostatic pressure	Local
Lymphatic obstruction	Lymphatic obstruction	Local
Generalized		
Congestive cardiac failure	Increased venous hydrostatic pressure, renal salt and water retention	Jugular veins (intravascular, not 'oedema'), lower limb, pulmonary
Cirrhosis	Decreased plasma oncotic pressure, renal salt and water retention, increased venous hydrostatic pressure	Ascites, lower limb
Nephrotic syndrome	Decreased plasma oncotic pressure, renal salt and water retention	Facial, lower limb
Septicaemia	Capillary leak	Lower limb, pulmonary
Allergic reactions (angio-oedema)	Capillary leak	Facial
Cyclical ('idiopathic')	?	Lower limb
Drugs	Increased venous hydrostatic pressure, renal salt and water retention	Lower limb

Under normal circumstances, protein is largely excluded from glomerular filtrate by an intact GCW. As shown in Fig. 6.2, the GCW comprises three layers: the endothelial cell, the GBM and the visceral glomerular epithelial cell (GEC). Each layer appears to act as a barrier to filtration of protein, but this function is subserved predominantly by the GBM and by the slit pore between cytoplasmic extensions ('foot processes' or 'podocytes') of the GEC. The visceral GEC can be visualized as a small-headed octopus with its many discrete feet (podocytes) draped over and covering the outer surface of each glomerular loop. Between the podocytes are slit pores, across which are spread thin diaphragms consisting of newly recognized proteins such as nephrin. Mutations of various podocyte proteins including nephrin have been identified as causing familial nephrotic syndrome, and their identification has brought an understanding of the molecular structure of the slit diaphragm and podocyte–GBM interactions.

The GBM also consists of specialized structural proteins, including certain collagens and charged heparin-like molecules. These molecules are arranged so that discrete pores prevent movement of large molecules (size selectivity) and charged ions (charge selectivity) across the GBM. Thus albumin, which is negatively charged and has a molecular weight of 67 000 D, does not pass across the normal GBM. Haemoglobin has a similar molecular weight to albumin but is not charged; therefore when it is released from red blood cells (haemolysis), it can pass across the GBM and is excreted in the urine (haemoglobinuria). Smaller proteins such as myoglobin (17,000 D) and monomeric light chains (22 000 D) pass across freely, whereas larger molecules such as ferritin (480 000 D) may only pass across severely disrupted GBMs.

Although the mesangial cell is not anatomically part of the GCW, it can alter the filtration of proteins because of its contractile properties (which alter the surface area of GCW available for filtration) and its ability to absorb, metabolize and discharge macromolecules into renal lymphatic channels.

Normal and abnormal proteinuria

Normal urine contains a small amount of protein, less than 150 mg/day in adults. Normal urinary protein consists of proteins of small molecular weight which have been filtered across the GCW and not reabsorbed by tubular cells, and proteins such as Tamm–Horsfall protein which are secreted by tubular cells. Heavy exercise, fever and prolonged standing ('orthostasis') may increase proteinuria in otherwise normal individuals. As explained above, larger proteins such as albumin are found in only small amounts in normal urine.

Abnormal proteinuria most commonly arises because of failure of the GCW filtration barrier ('glomerular proteinuria') but it can also result from decreased protein reabsorption into, or increased protein release from, tubular epithelial cells ('tubular proteinuria'; see Fig. 6.3). Tubular proteinuria consists of low molecular weight proteins (generally less than 40 000 D) and usually amounts to less than 1 g/day. Glomerular proteinuria consists of proteins of greater molecular size, and may be up to many grams per day. In some glomerular diseases in which the injury is of a limited nature, such as minimal change disease, protein loss into the urine is largely restricted to molecules the size of albumin or less ('selective proteinuria'), whereas with more extensive damage immunoglobulins and even larger proteins may be found in the urine ('nonselective proteinuria'). Note that even with glomerular proteinuria, the tubules do have some capacity to reabsorb a fraction of the filtered protein. When glomerular proteinuria is severe, nephrotic syndrome may develop, as occurred with the current patient.

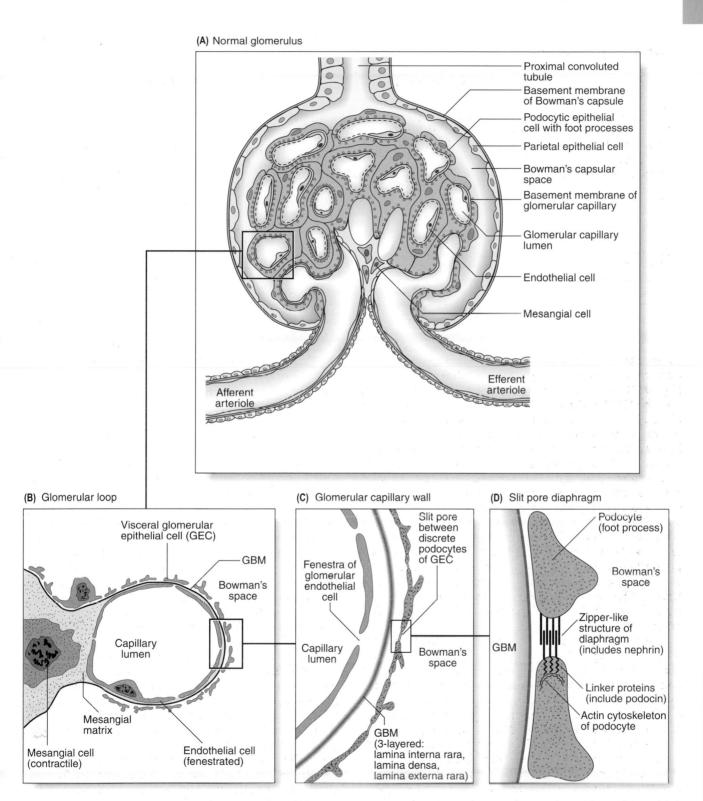

(A) Normal glomerulus

- Proximal convoluted tubule
- Basement membrane of Bowman's capsule
- Podocytic epithelial cell with foot processes
- Parietal epithelial cell
- Bowman's capsular space
- Basement membrane of glomerular capillary
- Glomerular capillary lumen
- Endothelial cell
- Mesangial cell

Efferent arteriole

Afferent arteriole

(B) Glomerular loop

- Visceral glomerular epithelial cell (GEC)
- GBM
- Bowman's space
- Capillary lumen
- Mesangial matrix
- Mesangial cell (contractile)
- Endothelial cell (fenestrated)

(C) Glomerular capillary wall

- Slit pore between discrete podocytes of GEC
- Fenestra of glomerular endothelial cell
- Capillary lumen
- Bowman's space
- GBM (3-layered: lamina interna rara, lamina densa, lamina externa rara)

(D) Slit pore diaphragm

- Podocyte (foot process)
- Bowman's space
- GBM
- Zipper-like structure of diaphragm (includes nephrin)
- Linker proteins (include podocin)
- Actin cytoskeleton of podocyte

Fig. 6.2 (A) Structure of the normal glomerulus, which is a capillary network fed by an afferent arteriole, and drained by an efferent arteriole; (B) glomerular loop, consisting of a capillary lumen lying beneath glomerular epithelial cells (GEC) and adjacent to mesangium; (C) glomerular capillary wall, comprising glomerular endothelial cells surrounded by the glomerular basement membrane (GBM) and GEC; (D) slit diaphragm of podocyte with newly-recognized structural and signalling proteins.

The principal causes of proteinuria are listed in Box 6.1. The most important of these in clinical terms are those conditions which cause damage to the glomerulus. Glomerular disease may be primary (glomerulonephritis) or secondary to systemic diseases such as diabetes mellitus. In addition, glomerular disease may occur as a component or consequence of widespread renal scarring which occurs late in the course of any chronic renal disease. In the latter situation the glomerular scarring is called 'glomerulosclerosis'.

See 6.1: 2.

Interesting facts

Urinary dipsticks are used in screening for proteinuria and differ in their specificity and sensitivity for albumin. Some are highly specific and able to detect albumin in low concentration ('microalbuminuria'). To quantitate protein excretion the urine sample needs to be collected over a specified period of time, or a factor introduced to take account of how concentrated the urinary sample is. Urinary creatinine concentration is a useful correction factor, because in an individual patient the daily excretion of creatinine tends to remain constant. Thus it is common practice to express urinary protein as a ratio to urinary creatinine.

Nephrotic syndrome

Clinical features

Nephrotic syndrome (or nephrosis) consists of a diagnostic triad of heavy proteinuria, which leads to

Normal **Tubular** **Glomerular**

➡ Large proteins   → Small proteins

Fig. 6.3 Proteinuria, occurring in normal kidneys or as a result of tubular or glomerular disease.

hypoalbuminaemia, which in turn causes oedema in a range of anatomical locations (Table 6.2 and Fig. 6.4).

Complications of nephrotic syndrome are relatively common, and their frequency increases with the severity

Box 6.1 Principal causes of proteinuria

Normal kidneys

Normal (<150 mg/24 h)
Exercise
Fever
Orthostasis

Abnormal kidneys

Tubular diseases (≤1 g/24 h)
Glomerular disease (>1 or 2 g/24 h)
    Primary glomerulonephritis
    Secondary glomerular disease in:
        systemic diseases such as diabetes mellitus,
        amyloidosis
        generalized renal scarring

Case 6.1 Proteinuria and the nephrotic syndrome: 2

Investigations

Kylie's GP organized some blood and urine tests. Her serum creatinine was normal, and serum albumin was very low at *13 g/L. Microscopic examination of spun urinary sediment was normal except for the presence of many hyaline (proteinaceous) casts. Urinary protein excretion was *6 g/day, and consisted mainly of albumin. Serum cholesterol was *9.6 mmol/L and serum triglycerides were normal.

When Kylie returned to be reviewed by her GP 2 days later, she had gained an extra 3 kg in weight and her oedema was worse. In addition, she was complaining of pain in her right calf, which appeared to be more swollen than the left. Her GP suspected a deep vein thrombosis in her right calf and treated her with anticoagulants.

In summary, the results of Kylie's tests indicated that her generalized oedema was caused by hypoalbuminaemia, which in turn was due to heavy proteinuria. As the proteinuria was predominantly albuminuria, it can be considered as 'selective', suggesting a restricted injury to the glomerular filtration barrier.

Her subsequent clinical course raises the following questions:

1. Why did the oedema progress?
2. Was the hypercholesterolaemia related to her renal disease?
3. What was the relationship between her renal disease and the deep venous thrombosis?

*Values outside normal range; see Appendix.

Table 6.2 Nephrotic syndrome

	Pathophysiology
Diagnostic triad	
Proteinuria >3.5 g/day	Disease of glomerular capillary wall
Serum albumin <30 g/L	Urinary protein loss
Oedema	Low plasma oncotic pressure
	Salt and water retention by kidneys
Complications	
Hypercholesterolaemia	Increased hepatic synthesis and reduced metabolism of lipoproteins
Thrombosis	Venous obstruction caused by oedema
	Increased hepatic synthesis of clotting factors
	Urinary loss of antithrombotic proteins
Infection	Urinary loss of immunoglobulins and other defence proteins
Kidney failure	Intravascular volume depletion (acute)
	Intrarenal oedema (acute)
	Primary renal disease causing glomerular damage
	Proteinuria causing interstitial inflammation and fibrosis
Malnutrition	Severe protein loss

of the proteinuria. Some of the complications arise because of loss of 'protective' factors in the urine, and others are caused by increased hepatic production of 'damaging' factors, apparently as part of a generalized compensatory hepatic synthetic response primarily involving albumin. The major complications of nephrosis and their pathogenesis are described in Table 6.2. These complications are clinically relevant and, in untreated nephrosis, have an important bearing on what happens to the patient. Chronic kidney disease may develop due to progression of the primary disease, or due to toxic effects of filtered protein which in large amounts may injure tubular cells or cause them to produce proinflammatory and profibrotic cytokines, leading to interstitial inflammation and fibrosis.

It has been established that this patient has severe nephrotic syndrome with complications. The next questions to be asked include the following.

- What type of kidney disease caused the nephrosis?
- Can and should the disease be treated?

These questions will be answered below. See 6.1: 3.

NEPHROTIC SYNDROME

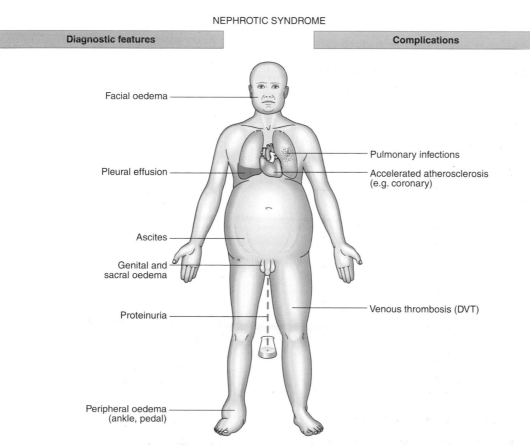

Fig. 6.4 Diagnostic clinical features and complications of nephrotic syndrome (representative site of complication shown, but may occur at multiple sites).

Renal biopsy

Percutaneous renal biopsy, in which a small specimen of kidney tissue is obtained under local anaesthesia using a specialized needle, can be used to establish diagnosis and prognosis in patients with suspected renal parenchymal disease, including those with nephrotic syndrome. Although it is a safe procedure, it can be complicated by bleeding and so is used selectively. It may not be used when the diagnosis is in little doubt, when it is unlikely to lead to a change in therapy, or when the chance of complication is greater than usual.

Case 6.1	Proteinuria and the nephrotic syndrome: 3

Diagnosis

Kylie was referred to a nephrologist to have a renal biopsy. However, the nephrologist informed Kylie's GP that in this particular instance there was no need to perform a renal biopsy as the clinical features and (subsequent) response to treatment predicted both diagnosis and prognosis with high sensitivity and specificity.

This portion of the patient's history raises the following questions:

1. How can the glomerular disease be diagnosed?
2. Is a kidney biopsy always necessary to make the diagnosis?

Renal biopsy specimens are examined by light microscopy with standard and special stains, by electron microscopy and by immunofluorescence microscopy. The main parameters examined are listed in Table 6.3. Abnormalities may be segmental (involving part of a glomerulus only) or global (the whole glomerulus), and focal (involving a few glomeruli only) or diffuse (most glomeruli).

The classification of glomerular disease depends largely on histopathological features of renal biopsy specimens. There are many types of glomerular disease, and the classification system is somewhat complicated and is revised every few years or so. Therefore, the student should not aim to become an expert. A basic understanding of how renal biopsies are examined and of a few important varieties of glomerular disease (described below and in Chapters 7 and 8) is sufficient for most non-nephrologists.

With minimal change disease, light and immunofluorescence microscopy are normal. The only abnormality is diffuse fusion or effacement of podocytes of the GEC seen on electron microscopy (Fig. 6.5). This occurs due to disruption of the actin cytoskeletal network of podocytes.

Causes of nephrotic syndrome

The main causes of nephrotic syndrome are listed in Table 6.4. The condition may arise as an isolated (primary) pathology, or as a component of a systemic disease.

In a child with new onset nephrotic syndrome and normal blood pressure, benign (or inactive) urinary sediment (see Chapter 7) and normal serum creatinine, minimal change disease is by far the most likely diagnosis. The patient's age and associated clinical features are very useful in predicting the diagnosis in other cases, though a renal biopsy would usually be performed. Membranous glomerulonephritis is the principal cause of nephrotic syndrome in adults. It usually occurs in isolation ('primary' or 'idiopathic'), but sometimes develops as a complication of diseases such as **systemic lupus erythematosus** or cancer. Focal sclerosing glomerulonephritis can occur in any age group.

Table 6.3 Renal biopsy: parameters

Light microscopy	
Glomerulus	Glomerular capillary wall thickness, cellularity, matrix, sclerosis
	Focal *versus* diffuse, segmental *versus* global
Blood vessels	Wall thickness, inflammation, occlusion
Tubule cells	Hypertrophy, atrophy
Interstitium	Inflammation, fibrosis
Electron microscopy	
Glomerular epithelial cell podocytes	Discrete *versus* fused
Glomerular basement membrane	Thickness, regularity
Site of electron-dense deposits	Mesangial, subendothelial, subepithelial
Immunofluorescence microscopy	
Glomerular pattern	Capillary wall *versus* mesangial, linear *versus* granular
Ligand of fluorescent antibody	Immunoglobulins, complement component, light chain

Fig 6.5 Electron micrograph of (A) normal glomerular capillary wall (GCW) and (B) GCW from a patient with minimal change disease showing extensive fusion of the foot processes (podocytes) of glomerular epithelial cells. C, capillary lumen; B, Bowman's space; *, basement membrane; arrow head, fenestrated glomerular endothelial cell; arrow, podocytes (which are normally discrete, but fused in minimal change disease); E, red blood cell.

Table 6.4 Major causes of nephrotic syndrome

	Usual age	Response to treatment	Risk of chronic kidney disease
Primary			
Minimal change disease	Child or adolescent	Yes	No
Focal sclerosing GN	Child or adolescent, adult, elderly	(Yes)	Yes
Membranous GN	Adult, elderly	(Yes)	Yes
Mesangiocapillary GN	Adult	Yes	Yes
Secondary			
Diabetic nephropathy	Adult, elderly	(No)	Yes
Amyloidosis	(Adult)*, elderly	(No)	Yes
Systemic lupus erythematosus	Adult, elderly	Yes	Yes

*Less frequent. Other parentheses indicate that this is sometimes the case. GN, glomerulonephritis.

Natural history and response to treatment

Treatment of nephrotic syndrome depends on the exact pathological diagnosis. In general, primary forms of glomerulonephritis causing nephrotic syndrome are treated with corticosteroids. These have an anti-inflammatory action involving depletion of T lymphocytes and impairment of polymorphonuclear leucocyte function. In some cases, immunosuppressive drugs such as cyclophosphamide are used. With secondary glomerulonephritis, treatment is directed towards the primary disease, though this may be modified considerably with renal involvement.

Response to treatment varies considerably depending on the diagnosis, as summarized in Table 6.4. Response is excellent with minimal change disease, but relapses are not infrequent. Response is much less predictable with other diagnoses. In the face of continuing nephrosis, the patient is at risk of developing complications (see Table 6.2), some of which can be prevented or treated.

Proteinuria and the nephrotic syndrome: 4

Treatment

Kylie was treated with corticosteroids and within a few weeks her nephrotic syndrome resolved completely. Two years later her disease relapsed, and once again she responded rapidly to corticosteroids. She has remained completely well since.

Interesting facts

Although the severity of proteinuria tends to predict the risk of complications of nephrosis, this is not always the case. For example, minimal change disease is unique in that chronic kidney disease does not develop, even when proteinuria is massive and unremitting. Thus kidney scarring in proteinuria is not just determined by the amount of filtered protein, but more by intrinsic properties of the particular protein and other proinflammatory and profibrotic events.

Without successful treatment, nephrotic syndrome will persist in most patients, with the attendant risk of complications. Only in minimal change disease is there no risk of developing chronic kidney disease (see 6.1: 4).

GLOMERULONEPHRITIS AND THE ACUTE NEPHRITIC SYNDROME

7

Chapter objectives

After studying this chapter you should be able to:

1. Describe the components of the acute nephritic syndrome and its variations.

2. Describe other forms of presentation of glomerulonephritis (GN).

3. Understand the pathogenesis of post-streptococcal GN.

4. Differentiate acute nephritis occurring with post-streptococcal GN, IgA disease and systemic diseases.

5. Discuss the consequences of glomerular disease.

6. Describe the parameters of urinary sediment examination.

7. Discuss the natural history of post-streptococcal GN.

Introduction

Acute glomerulonephritis (GN) refers generally to inflammatory renal diseases affecting the glomeruli of some or all of the million nephrons of each kidney. Although this classification is based largely on the pathological appearance of glomeruli, other components of the nephron, blood vessels and renal interstitium are involved to a variable extent. Many of the acute glomerulonephritides are primary or idiopathic, whereas with others a secondary cause is identified. The pathogenesis of GN varies with the diagnosis and may involve multiple factors. With many forms it is only partially understood. In this chapter, the pathogenesis of GN will be explained by a discussion of the presentation and diagnosis of a case of acute nephritic syndrome.

There are a bewildering number of types of primary and secondary GN, and the systems of classification are overlapping and confusing. For this reason, the student is urged to concentrate only on the common or classic forms of disease which are discussed in this chapter. See Case 7.1:1.

Urinary sediment examination

To confirm the presence of renal inflammation, sediment examination should be performed on a centrifuged sample of fresh urine. Every medical student and graduate should be confident in examining urinary sediment. To allow quantification of the urinary abnormalities, this should be done in a standardized fashion. Ten millilitres of urine is spun at $2500 \times g$ for 5 min, 9.5 mL of the urine is then discarded, the sediment is resuspended in the remaining 0.5 mL of urine by gentle tapping of the test tube, and this resuspended sediment is examined using a counting chamber. Normal urine may contain up to 500 red blood cells, 2000 white blood cells and 15 hyaline (but not granular or cellular) casts per millilitre.

The finding of an excess number of red or white cells may be explained by abnormalities anywhere in the urinary tract. It should be noted that a positive dipstick test for blood indicates the presence of haem pigment, whereas microscopy is required to confirm the presence of red blood cells (this is discussed in more detail in Chapter 10). When cells or cellular debris aggregate in the tubular lumen, they may form casts of the tubule. Granular or cellular (epithelial, red or white cell) casts indicate the presence of renal parenchymal disease, whereas hyaline (proteinaceous) casts are found with proteinuria. An 'active' sediment contains elements consistent with renal inflammation and/or cell necrosis, whereas a 'benign' sediment may contain a few cells and only hyaline casts. Fresh urine should be examined as casts may break down within 1–2 h. Figure 7.1 shows examples of urinary casts. See Case 7.1:2.

Interesting facts

Healthy individuals pass on average up to two million erythrocytes in their urine per day, with the actual number in an individual varying from 4 fold less to more than this. These cells generally come from the kidney, and are thus 'dysmorphic' in appearance. As urinary dipsticks for haem pigment can detect as few as 5–20 erythrocytes per microlitre, normal urinary blood should usually not be detectable by dipstick testing.

Case 7.1 Glomerulonephritis and the acute nephritic syndrome: 1

Nephritic syndrome

Michael Willandra is a 22-year-old Aboriginal Australian who presented to the local hospital of a western New South Wales town complaining of headache and dark urine. He had also noticed a reduction in urine output (oliguria) even though he had a normal fluid intake. In the past Michael had had frequent sore throats and skin infections. Approximately 2 weeks before presentation he had had another sore throat which resolved spontaneously after 8 days. The resident doctor noted that he had facial swelling and a blood pressure of 165/105. His jugular venous pressure was raised 2 cm and rales (sounds produced by passage of air through fluid in the lower respiratory tract) were heard on auscultation at the bases of both lungs. There was a creamy exudate on his tonsils and mild pharyngeal erythema. Dipstick analysis of urine revealed blood and protein. The doctor suspected that Michael had acute GN.

The important clinical features in this patient include the occurrence of oliguria, dark urine, hypertension and fluid overload 2 weeks after a sore throat. The questions that arise from this clinical history include the following:

1. What is the pathophysiology of each of the clinical features?
2. Are the clinical features interrelated?
3. What is the relationship of the sore throat to the acute illness which followed 2 weeks later?
4. What made the doctor suspect a diagnosis of GN?

The answers to these questions will be revealed in the initial sections of this chapter. Before this, however, we must discuss the examination of urinary sediment, the first and one of the most important tests in a suspected case of renal disease, which provides a non-invasive glimpse of the inflammatory processes which occur within the kidney.

(A)   (B)

Fig. 7.1 Urinary casts: (A) hyaline, (B) red cell. Casts form within the tubular lumen and therefore take on the shape of the lumen with parallel sides. Photographs courtesy of Prof. J. Lawrence.

Case 7.1 Glomerulonephritis and the acute nephritic syndrome: 2

Initial investigations

Urinary sediment examination showed more than *100 red cells per microlitre, as well as a moderate number of white cell and red cell casts. Serum creatinine was elevated at *0.16 mmol/L. Based on this the doctor told Michael he had 'nephritis'.

The obvious question to be asked at this stage is: which of the clinical and laboratory features of the patient are diagnostic, characteristic or consistent with the nephritic syndrome (or nephritis)?

*Values outside the normal range; see Appendix.

Box 7.1 Presentation of glomerular disease

Nephritic syndrome*
Nephrotic syndrome†
Asymptomatic proteinuria and/or microscopic haematuria
Macroscopic haematuria
Acute kidney injury (acute renal failure)
Progressive chronic kidney disease
Hypertension

*Haematuria, hypertension, renal functional impairment and oliguria.
†Heavy proteinuria, hypoalbuminaemia and oedema.

Presentation and consequences of glomerular disease

Patients with glomerular disease may present in a number of different ways; these are listed in Box 7.1. The spectrum of presentation includes asymptomatic microscopic haematuria and/or proteinuria discovered on routine medical check, acute or chronic kidney disease, hypertension, or full blown (or a limited form of) nephrotic or nephritic syndromes. The nephrotic syndrome is described in Chapter 6.

The nephritic syndrome consists of haematuria, hypertension and renal functional impairment (reduced glomerular filtration rate (GFR), reflected by the raised serum creatinine), as was found in the present case.

The haematuria and active urinary sediment are indicative of renal inflammation; oliguria and renal functional impairment are a consequence of glomerular infiltration with inflammatory cells and release of vasoactive hormones and cytokines; and hypertension is the result of salt and water retention and vasoactive hormone release.

The consequences of glomerular disease and the underlying pathophysiology of each feature are described in Table 7.1. Renal functional impairment in glomerular disease is multifactorial and arises because of the acute inflammatory process (proliferation of intrinsic glomerular cells, glomerular infiltration with leucocytes and haemodynamic changes induced by vasoactive hormones and cytokines) and chronic renal scarring (caused by continuing inflammation, hypertension, proteinuria and other factors). Hypertension occurs in acute nephritis because of salt and water retention (a consequence of the reduction of GFR), glomerular capillary and arteriolar scarring, and neurohumoral changes, in particular activation of the renin–angiotensin system.

Table 7.1 Consequences of glomerular disease

Feature	Pathophysiology
Proteinuria	Impaired filtration barrier function of GCW
Haematuria	Leak into Bowman's space across GCW or into tubular lumen
Renal impairment	Structural and/or functional damage to glomeruli and tubulointerstitium
Hypertension	Salt and water retention, activation of the renin–angiotensin system

GCW, glomerular capillary wall.

The diagnosis of glomerular disease and, specifically, the nephritic syndrome can almost always be established by a combination of clinical features, serological tests and renal biopsy. This was the case with the current patient. These clinical and laboratory features also give clues to the pathogenesis of the disease and its complications. See Case 7.1:3.

Investigation of glomerulonephritis

There are a number of serological tests which are useful for establishing, confirming or supporting a specific diagnosis in patients with GN (Table 7.2). A positive test result suggests the primary diagnosis but does not prove that it is the cause of the renal disease. Some of these serological abnormalities are actually involved in the pathogenesis of the renal lesion, and will be discussed in more detail later in this chapter.

Renal biopsy usually establishes the diagnosis definitively. The components of renal biopsy examination are discussed in Chapter 6 (see Table 6.3). In the current patient the history, positive ASOT, low serum C3 and renal biopsy appearances were all consistent with a diagnosis of post-streptococcal GN.

Differential diagnosis of acute glomerulonephritis

GN may occur in isolation or as part of a multisystem disease. Amongst diseases in which GN is the sole manifestation, a specific precipitant is recognized in only a few. In the current case, the precipitant was a streptococcal throat infection occurring 2 weeks before the onset of GN. This once common disease is seen less frequently nowadays, except in underprivileged populations. The streptococcal infection may also be a skin infection. A similar type of GN can be seen following bacterial infections of other types (postinfectious GN). Many patients presenting with other types of GN give a history of a respiratory illness in the preceding days to weeks. Only in some patients is the respiratory illness of definite pathogenetic significance. A common form of GN that needs to be distinguished from post-streptococcal GN is IgA disease (or mesangial IgA nephropathy). IgA disease is a common type of GN, characterized by acute nephritis and, in particular, macroscopic haematuria occurring at the time or within a few days of a viral sore throat. The shorter prodrome and its frequently recurrent nature help to distinguish it at presentation from post-streptococcal GN (Table 7.3 and Fig. 7.3).

Acute nephritic syndrome can occur in a number of conditions that are either restricted to the kidney or involve multiple organs (systemic diseases). Some of the

---

Case 7.1 Glomerulonephritis and the acute nephritic syndrome: 3

Diagnostic investigations

The history of a sore throat 14 days before the onset of acute nephritis was consistent with a diagnosis of post-streptococcal GN. Serum antistreptococcal O titre (ASOT) was elevated and serum concentration of the third complement component (C3) was low, indicating complement activation, and was consistent with the presumed diagnosis. In this disease, the renal lesion represents an immunological reaction to nephritogenic antigens in the microorganism responsible for the sore throat.

The patient was referred to a nephrologist who arranged a renal biopsy (Fig. 7.2). On light microscopy, all glomeruli were infiltrated with neutrophil leucocytes and there was proliferation of mesangial and endothelial cells. Electron microscopy showed large electron-dense deposits lying between the podocytes of the visceral glomerular epithelial cells and the glomerular basement

membrane. Immunofluorescence microscopy was positive for IgM, IgA and C3 in a granular capillary wall pattern. (A renal biopsy is frequently not necessary in this situation because the clinical and other laboratory features can be highly suggestive of the diagnosis and the long-term prognosis is usually good.)

The results of these diagnostic investigations lead to several questions which will be answered in the following sections of this chapter:

1. Which serological tests are necessary to establish the diagnosis and classification of GN?
2. Which renal biopsy features are useful or necessary to classify GN?
3. What insights do these features give to the pathogenesis of the renal lesion?

(A)

(C)

Fig. 7.2 Renal biopsy of the patient with post-streptococcal glomerulonephritis. (A) Light microscopy showing proliferation of intrinsic glomerular cells and infiltrating neutrophil leucocytes. (B) Electron microscopy showing large immune deposits ('humps' H) projecting into the Bowman's space (B) between the glomerular basement membrane (*) and glomerular epithelial cell (arrows). (C) Immunofluorescence microscopy showing coarse granular pattern for IgG along the glomerular capillary wall.

Table 7.2 Important diagnostic serological tests for glomerulonephritis

Test	Diagnosis
Serum complement	
Low C3	Post-streptococcal GN, mesangiocapillary GN
Low C3 and C4	Systemic lupus erythematosus
Others	
ANA, anti-double-stranded DNA antibody	Systemic lupus erythematosus
ANCA	Microscopic polyangiitis or Wegener's granulomatosis
Anti-GBM antibody	Goodpasture's syndrome
ASOT	Post-streptococcal GN
HBsAg	Hepatitis B
Anti-HCV	Hepatitis C
HIV	AIDS
VDRL	Syphilis

ANA, antinuclear antibody; ANCA, antineutrophil cytoplasmic antibody; ASOT, antistreptococcal O titre; GBM, glomerular basement membrane; HBsAg, hepatitis B surface antigen; HCV, hepatitis C virus; VDRL, Venereal Disease Research Laboratory (serological test for syphilis).

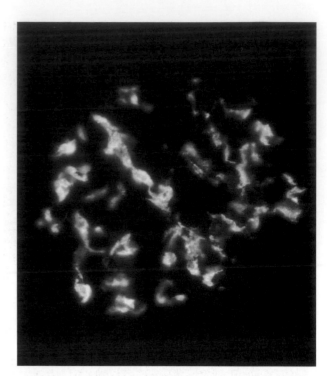

Fig. 7.3 Immunofluorescence of renal biopsy from a patient with IgA disease, showing positive immunofluorescence for IgA in a mesangial distribution. Contrast this with the 'capillary wall' distribution in Figs 7.2 (C) and 7.4.

Table 7.3 Clinical and pathological differences between post-streptococcal glomerulonephritis (GN) and IgA disease

	Post-streptococcal GN	IgA disease
Antecedent pharyngitis	Yes, 10–14 days	Yes, 0–4 days
Acute nephritis	Yes	Yes
Other presentations	No	Yes*
Recurrence	No	Yes
Long-term prognosis	Excellent	Variable
Diagnostic tests		
Serological	Low C3, positive ASOT	–
Renal biopsy	Glomerular neutrophil infiltration (LM)	Mesangial IgA (IF)†
	Subepithelial electron-dense deposits (EM)	Mesangial electron-dense deposits (EM)

ASOT, antistreptococcal O titre; LM, light microscopy; EM, electron microscopy; IF, immunofluorescence microscopy.
*Other presentations of IgA disease include macroscopic haematuria, nephrosis (uncommon), hypertension, chronic kidney disease.
†See Fig. 7.3.

Box 7.2 Important causes of acute nephritic syndrome

Primary
Post-streptococcal glomerulonephritis
Postinfective glomerulonephritis
IgA disease*
Mesangiocapillary (membranoproliferative) glomerulonephritis
Crescentic glomerulonephritis

Secondary to systemic disease
Systemic lupus erythematosus
Microscopic polyangiitis and Wegener's granulomatosis

*Can present less commonly as a systemic vasculitis with skin, joint, gastrointestinal and renal involvement (Henoch–Schönlein purpura).

important examples are listed in Box 7.2. Amongst these, IgA disease is the only common disease. Nevertheless, it is important to consider the other conditions because, without rapid treatment, irreversible renal failure may develop. Rapidly progressive GN, in which renal failure develops over a period of days to weeks, is characteristic of several of these conditions, including primary crescentic GN, microscopic polyangiitis and Goodpasture's syndrome.

(A)   (B)

Fig. 7.4 Immunofluorescence pattern of renal biopsy specimen of glomerulonephritis initiated by: (A) autoimmune response to glomerular antigen (linear), and (B) immune response to circulating or planted extrarenal antigen (granular). Half of the glomerulus in (A) is replaced by a glomerular crescent which is not immunofluorescent. In both (A) and (B) the immunofluorescence is in a glomerular capillary wall distribution.

Interesting facts

IgA disease is the most common form of GN worldwide. Its presentation is very variable, ranging from isolated microscopic haematuria to (rarely) a rapidly progressive GN. Although the clinical course is benign in the majority of patients, IgA disease is so common that it is (after diabetes) the second most frequent condition causing endstage kidney disease.

Pathogenesis of acute glomerulonephritis

Current classification systems for GN are confusing, which is not surprising given the incomplete knowledge of pathogenesis and the overlapping morphological characteristics of many types of GN.

GN may be initiated by an immune response to an exogenous antigen such as a microbial product (including streptococcal products as in the current case) or to an endogenous antigen (such as DNA with systemic lupus erythematosus; SLE). Less commonly, it may be initiated by an autoimmune response to a renal antigen, such as a component of the glomerular basement membrane in Goodpasture's syndrome (Figs. 7.4A and 7.5). The antibodies involved in these responses may form the basis for diagnostic serological tests for these diseases (see Table 7.2). A number of other effector mechanisms involving leucocytes, platelets, complement, coagulation factors and humoral products of intrinsic and infiltrating cells, act in concert with these immune mechanisms to cause glomerular injury.

When the antigen forms part of a circulating immune complex or is deposited in the kidney (e.g. on the glomerular capillary wall) to form an immune complex *in situ*, the immunofluorescence pattern is discontinuous or granular (Fig. 7.4B). In this case, corresponding electron-dense deposits are seen with electron microscopy. This pattern is seen, for example, in membranous GN, post-streptococcal GN and SLE. In most cases it is unclear whether the immune complex forms primarily in the circulation or in the kidney.

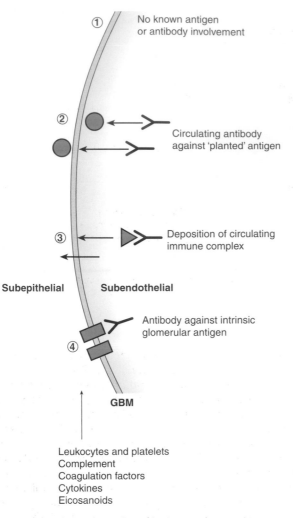

① No known antigen
or antibody involvement

② Circulating antibody
against 'planted' antigen

③ Deposition of circulating
immune complex

Subepithelial   **Subendothelial**

Antibody against intrinsic
glomerular antigen

④

GBM

Leukocytes and platelets
Complement
Coagulation factors
Cytokines
Eicosanoids

Fig. 7.5 Schematic representation of immunopathogenetic mechanisms of acute glomerulonephritis and the influence of other cellular and humoral mediators. Antigens may be deposited on the glomerular basement membrane before antibody deposition or as part of circulating antigen–antibody complexes, or may be self-antigens (usually modified) in the glomerular basement membrane.

Fig. 7.6 Cellular crescent (*) occupying three-quarters of the circumference of a glomerulus and compressing the glomerular tuft.

In contrast, when the antibody is directed against an intrinsic renal antigen, the immunofluorescence pattern is continuous or linear, as seen in Goodpasture's syndrome (Fig. 7.4A). In the latter situation, there should be no electron-dense deposits seen with electron microscopy.

Whether or not immune complex formation leads to the development of GN depends on numerous factors, including the nature of the antigen, the size of the complex, the antibody, the clearance of complexes by phagocytic cells, and other glomerular haemodynamic, cellular and humoral influences (Fig. 7.5).

Pathology of acute glomerulonephritis

The glomerulus may be altered in a limited number of ways in GN. Intrinsic cells (endothelial, mesangial and epithelial) may proliferate; circulating leucocytes may infiltrate; platelets may accumulate; mesangial matrix may expand; the glomerular basement membrane may change; and scarring may develop.

A hallmark of severe disease is the development of a glomerular crescent, which is a cellular, fibrinous and, later, fibrous lesion in Bowman's space, arising from proliferation of extracapillary cells, including glomerular epithelial cells and macrophages (Fig 7.6). The greater the size and the number of crescents, the more severe the disease. Crescents may be seen in many forms of GN and, when large and numerous (in more than 50% of glomeruli), they are associated with a rapidly progressive clinical course in certain forms of vasculitis and in primary crescentic GN (see Table 7.4).

Outcome of glomerulonephritis

Given the fact that glomerulonephritides presenting with an acute nephritic picture may have a guarded prognosis, it is logical to ask about the natural history in this particular patient, and whether treatment could alter the clinical course. See 7.1: 4.

Table 7.4 Important types of glomerulonephritis (GN) and their usual clinical picture

Presentation	Primary	Secondary
Nephrotic syndrome	Minimal change disease Membranous nephropathy Focal sclerosing GN Mesangiocapillary GN	Diabetes mellitus[*] Amyloidosis[*] Systemic lupus erythematosus
Acute nephritic syndrome	Postinfectious GN Post-streptococcal GN IgA disease Mesangiocapillary GN	Systemic lupus erythematosus
Rapidly progressive GN	Crescentic GN	Microscopic polyangiitis Wegener's granulomatosis Goodpasture's syndrome

Asymptomatic haematuria/proteinuria can occur with almost all listed conditions.
[*]These conditions are associated with a non-inflammatory glomerulopathy rather than a true glomerulonephritis.

<table>
<tr><td>Case
7.1</td><td>**Glomerulonephritis and the acute nephritic syndrome: 4**</td></tr>
</table>

Outcome

The patient received antihypertensive therapy and a loop diuretic to control fluid accumulation. Within a period of weeks his serum creatinine returned to normal, and his oedema and hypertension resolved. After 6 months his urinary sediment was inactive.

Thus, the patient's acute nephritis settled without specific treatment of the renal inflammation. But does this apply to other forms of acute nephritis?

The outcome of acute GN varies greatly with the type of disease. In diseases in which the inciting antigen or event disappears spontaneously (as in the current case) or with treatment, the renal disease may resolve. In some circumstances, such as IgA disease and SLE, the disease may smoulder on or recur. When the disease remains active, smoulders on or recurs, the tendency is for progressive kidney scarring and kidney failure to occur over a variable period of time.

Clinicopathological correlations in glomerulonephritis

No current system of classification lends itself ideally to the study of GN and so understanding the condition can be a daunting task. Thus, medical students should limit their study to the most common and/or clinically important diseases. These are listed in Table 7.4.

Some primary and secondary glomerulonephritides are usually associated with the nephrotic syndrome, as discussed in Chapter 6. Other forms of glomerulonephritis, such as postinfectious GN and IgA disease, may present with an acute nephritic syndrome, while others, such as SLE and mesangiocapillary GN, may present with either acute nephritis or nephrosis. In the context of an acute nephritic presentation, clinical clues should be sought to the presence of an underlying systemic condition (see Fig. 7.7). As mentioned above, it is important to recognize the rare cases of rapidly progressive GN as they require emergency treatment.

Some important diagnostic features of the glomerular pathology in these diseases are listed in Table 7.5. These characteristic morphological and immunological features are sufficient to allow a definitive histological diagnosis to be made in the majority of cases. Further discussion of each condition included in Table 7.5 is beyond the scope of this text.

Interesting facts

Rapidly progressive GN is a rare medical emergency. It can occur as a primary kidney disease or as part of a systemic illness such as Wegener's granulomatosis, microscopic polyangiitis, Goodpasture's syndrome and, rarely, Henoch–Schönlein purpura (a multisystem variant of IgA disease) or SLE. It is characterized clinically by a nephritic picture with a rising serum creatinine, and histologically by the presence of glomerular crescents. With appropriate early treatment the disease may be halted or even cured; without treatment endstage kidney failure occurs quickly.

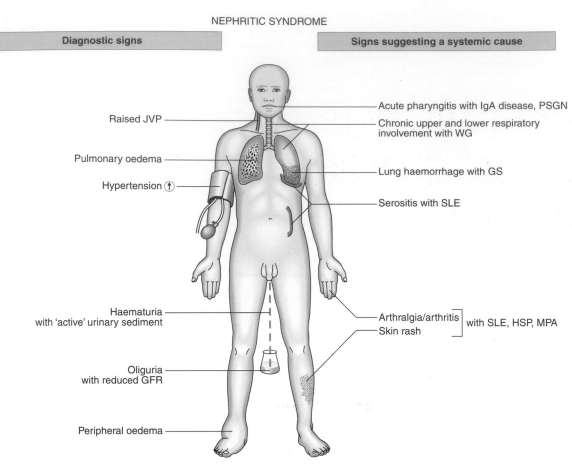

NEPHRITIC SYNDROME

Diagnostic signs

Signs suggesting a systemic cause

Raised JVP

Pulmonary oedema

Hypertension ⬆

Haematuria
with 'active' urinary sediment

Oliguria
with reduced GFR

Peripheral oedema

Acute pharyngitis with IgA disease, PSGN

Chronic upper and lower respiratory involvement with WG

Lung haemorrhage with GS

Serositis with SLE

Arthralgia/arthritis
Skin rash } with SLE, HSP, MPA

Fig. 7.7 Signs diagnostic of nephritic syndrome or suggestive of an underlying systemic condition. JVP, jugular venous pressure; PSGN, post-streptococcal glomerulonephritis; WG, Wegener's granulomatosis; GS, Goodpasture's syndrome; SLE, systemic lupus erythematosus; HSP, Henoch–Schönlein purpura; MPA, microscopic polyarteritis.

Table 7.5 Principal diagnostic glomerular appearances of important types of glomerulonephritis (GN)

	Light microscopy	*Electron microscopy*	*Immunofluorescence*
Minimal change disease	Normal	Diffuse foot process fusion	Negative
Membranous nephropathy	Thick GCW without glomerular hypercellularity	Subepithelial EDD ('lumps')	Finely granular, CW
Focal sclerosing GN	Focal segmental GS	Diffuse foot process fusion	IgM (segmental)
Mesangiocapillary GN	Thick GCW with glomerular hypercellularity	Subendothelial EDD, mesangial interposition	CW Ig and C
Postinfectious/ post-streptococcal GN	Hypercellular glomerulus	Subepithelial EDD ('humps')	CW Ig and C3
IgA disease	Mesangial proliferation	Mesangial EDD	Mesangial IgA
Diabetes mellitus	GS	Thick GBM, mesangial expansion	CW pseudolinear
Amyloidosis	Variable Negative birefringence with Congo Red stain	Amyloid fibrils	–
Systemic lupus erythematosus	Various patterns	EDD – multiple sites	CW and mesangial, Ig, C3,C1q
Rapidly progressive GN	Crescents	Variable	CW negative or granular or linear

C, complement; CW, capillary wall; EDD, electron-dense deposits; GBM, glomerular basement membrane; GCW, glomerular capillary wall; GS, glomerular sclerosis.

DIABETIC NEPHROPATHY AND CHRONIC KIDNEY DISEASE

8

Chapter objectives

After studying this chapter you should be able to:

1. Understand the natural history of diabetic nephropathy.

2. Discuss the common causes of chronic kidney disease (CKD).

3. Describe the presentation and natural history of CKD.

4. Appreciate the progressive nature of CKD.

5. Discuss the main consequences of CKD and their pathogenesis.

6. Understand the principles of treatment of patients with CKD.

Introduction

Diabetes mellitus, both insulin- and non-insulin-dependent, is an increasingly common cause of chronic kidney disease (CKD). For example, in Australia, which has very reliable national statistics on **end-stage kidney disease (ESKD)**, it now accounts for more than 30% of patients commencing dialysis or receiving a renal transplant. The incidence of diabetic nephropathy as a cause of ESKD is similar in Europe and even higher in New Zealand and the USA. In some ethnic groups, including Maoris, the incidence is more than 40%.

Whatever the cause of CKD, once a certain level of kidney dysfunction has been reached, kidney disease tends to progress towards end-stage. We understand some, but not all, of the reasons for this progression. Kidney failure has effects on almost all organ systems of the body and, as kidney dysfunction progresses, so these effects take on more clinical significance.

In this chapter we will discuss CKD and its consequences using an illustrative case of progressive kidney failure due to diabetic nephropathy. See Case 8.1:1.

Presentation of chronic kidney disease

The development of diabetic kidney disease in this patient was not surprising, as she already manifested other evidence of diabetic microvascular complications in the form of diabetic retinopathy requiring laser photocoagulation. Microvascular complications tend to affect multiple organs concomitantly, and it would be uncommon for a patient to develop diabetic retinopathy without coexisting nephropathy. Thus, in this patient the presentation is typical of someone with diabetes mellitus as the cause of CKD. By the time her serum creatinine was measured, she already had moderate kidney failure. However, a diagnosis of CKD may be made at any time during the course of the disease. This may range from early in an asymptomatic patient following the detection of serum biochemical or urinary abnormalities to very late in a patient with few symptoms. The range of presentations of CKD is shown in Box 8.1.

Note that in this patient there were several clinical features suggesting that salt and water were being retained as a consequence of low glomerular filtration rate (GFR). Thus, hypertension, raised jugular venous pressure, pulmonary rales and oedema were manifestations of expanded extracellular fluid and plasma volumes. Another factor contributing to her oedema was hypoalbuminaemia resulting from heavy proteinuria (see Chapter 6).

The natural history of CKD tends to vary according to the aetiology. For example, the typical clinical course for a patient with insulin-dependent diabetes mellitus (IDDM, or type 1 diabetes) who develops CKD (as some 40% do) is illustrated in Fig. 8.1. After about 5 years of IDDM, microalbuminuria develops (albumin excretion below the range usually detected by dipstick urinalysis).

Case 8.1 **Diabetic nephropathy and CKD: 1**

Diabetes mellitus and renal impairment

Raylene Tomlein is a 35-year-old woman who has had insulin-dependent diabetes mellitus since the age of 23 years. At age 30 years diabetic retinopathy was first diagnosed and she has received regular laser photocoagulation for this since then. She first noticed mild ankle swelling at age 32 years and this slowly increased in severity. For 2 years before the current presentation she had been on antihypertensives. Her blood pressure was 155/90. There was mild peripheral oedema and her jugular venous pressure wave was visible 3 cm above the clavicle at 45°. There were bibasal pulmonary rales. Otherwise, her physical examination was normal.

Urinalysis was positive for protein (+++) and blood (trace). Urinary protein excretion was *4.5 g/24 h. Serum creatinine was elevated at *0.29 mmol/L. Ultrasound examination showed echogenic kidneys of symmetrically reduced bipolar length.

This patient had clinical features (oedema, hypertension) which suggested that her kidney disease may have been present for at least 2 years. This raises the following important questions:

1. How can we differentiate acute kidney injury from CKD?
2. How does CKD present?
3. What is the significance of her other clinical features, namely diabetic retinopathy, hypertension and proteinuria?

These issues will be discussed below.

*Values outside normal range; see Appendix.

Box 8.1 Presentations of CKD

Asymptomatic serum biochemical abnormality
Asymptomatic proteinuria/haematuria
Hypertension
Symptomatic primary disease
Symptomatic uraemia
Complications of CKD

Overt proteinuria then develops over the next few years followed by progressive renal impairment which leads, after another 5 years or so, to ESKD. The course tends not to be quite as predictable in patients with non-insulin dependent diabetes mellitus (NIDDM, or type 2 diabetes).

Fig. 8.1 Typical clinical course of patient with insulin-dependent diabetes mellitus who develops nephropathy, from the onset of diabetes. *Proteinuria often falls late in CKD as glomerular filtration rate becomes severely impaired.

Table 8.1 Differentiation of acute and chronic kidney disease

	Acute	*Chronic*
History	Short (days–weeks)	Long (months–years)
Haemoglobin concentration	Normal	Low
Renal size	Normal	Reduced
Renal osteodystrophy*	Absent	Present
Peripheral neuropathy†	Absent	Present

*Osteodystrophy is bone disease.
†Peripheral neuropathy is disease or dysfunction of nerves supplying the limbs and peripheral tissues.

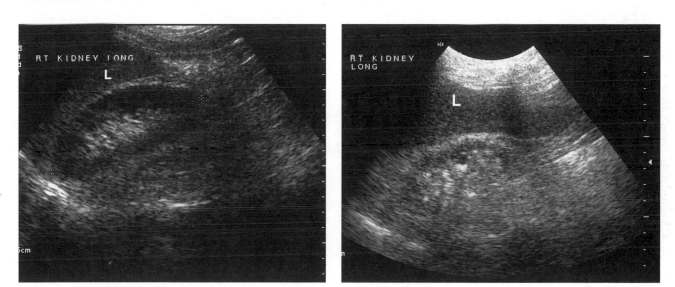

(A)   (B)

Fig. 8.2 Renal ultrasonography is useful in differentiating acute and chronic kidney disease. (A) Normal-sized kidney of acute kidney injury. Note that the normal kidney appears darker (less echogenic) than the adjacent liver (L). The kidney is 10.95 cm in bipolar length between markers. (B) Small, echogenic kidney of severe CKD. Note that a scarred kidney is brighter (more echogenic) than normal, and therefore less easy to distinguish from surrounding structures. The kidney is 7.36 cm in bipolar length.

Differentiating acute and chronic kidney disease

Kidney failure is defined as a reduced GFR, which causes the kidneys to lose the ability to excrete nitrogenous wastes such as urea and creatinine; this leads to an increase in their concentration in the serum (uraemia). Certain clues help to differentiate an acute reversible increase in serum creatinine concentration (acute kidney injury) from a chronic irreversible rise (CKD) (see Chapter 5 and Table 8.1). In the current patient, the long history and the reduction in renal size on ultrasonography (Fig. 8.2) indicate a chronic process. Similarly, a low haemoglobin concentration is typical of chronic rather than acute kidney disease.

Stages of chronic kidney disease

CKD may be divided into different stages depending on the GFR (Table 8.2). The functional changes need to be present for at least 3 months to indicate that the disease is chronic. Although arbitrary, such a division is useful in that it predicts the severity of clinical and biochemical derangements.

A patient may present at any stage of the disease. When the GFR is only mildly reduced (for example, greater than 60 mL/min) and the disease is not clearly progressive, a term such as mild kidney impairment may be used. ESKD, on the other hand, may be defined by the need for dialysis therapy or renal transplantation to sustain life (see Chapter 9).

Causes of chronic kidney disease

The major causes of ESKD are listed in Table 8.3. Diabetes mellitus (as in the current patient) is the most common cause. Glomerulonephritis forms the second largest group, and, amongst the glomerulonephritides, IgA disease is the commonest variant causing ESKD in most western communities, accounting for 25% of cases in this category. In the tropics, chronic obstruction due to renal calculi is a relatively common cause of CKD. Amongst elderly patients, CKD caused by renovascular disease is being diagnosed more frequently.

Interesting facts

Currently there are more than two million people worldwide with end-stage kidney disease (ESKD), and this number is predicted to more than double over the next decade.

The increase in patients with ESKD is being driven largely by the increased incidence of diabetes. In 2000 there were 150 million people worldwide with diabetes, one third in developed countries. It is estimated that by 2025 the number of diabetics will double, with a 30% increase in developed countries and a 130% increase in developing countries.

Interesting facts

Thirty years ago analgesic nephropathy was the second most common cause of ESKD in Australia (after glomerulonephritis), accounting for one quarter of cases. Due to legislation outlawing the sale of compound analgesics since 1980, it now accounts for less than 2% of new cases.

Pathology of diabetic nephropathy and chronic kidney disease

The renal pathological features of CKD consist of a mixture of changes typical of the primary disease and those which are common to CKD of all types. As the disease progresses, the disease-specific changes become less obvious and, in kidneys from patients with advanced disease, the histopathological changes become non-specific.

Early diagnostic changes in diabetic nephropathy include glomerular basement membrane thickening and expansion of the mesangium, and hyaline thickening of the afferent and efferent arterioles (Fig. 8.3). Usually there is superimposed hypertensive and sometimes infective damage (thickening of small arteries and arterioles, and interstitial inflammatory cells and scarring, respectively).

Table 8.3 Common causes of ESKD

	*Percentage incidence
Diabetes mellitus	30
Glomerulonephritis	25
Hypertension	15
Polycystic kidney disease	5
Vesicoureteric reflux	5
Unknown	5
Other	15

*Approximate incidence in Australia and New Zealand (source ANZDATA Registry, 2003–2006): these are representative of data for other developed countries.

Table 8.2 Stages of CKD

Stage of CKD	GFR* (mL/min)	Symptoms of uraemia or its complications	Serum biochemical derangements	Comment
1. Normal GFR†	>90	None	None	Not clearly progressive
2. Mild	60–90	None	Subtle	Early bone disease commences; increased risk of vascular disease
3. Moderate	30–60	Mild	Mild	Anaemia develops
4. Severe	15–30	Moderate	Moderate	Salt and water retention evident
5. End-stage	<5–15	Severe	Severe	Dialysis or renal transplantation necessary

*See Chapter 5 for a discussion of normal GFR (approximately 100 mL/min) and how it is affected by age, sex and body weight. The change in GFR needs to be present for at least 3 months.

†But with abnormal proteinuria, urine sediment and/or blood pressure.

Advanced CKD is characterized by progressive scarring of glomeruli (glomerulosclerosis) and tubulointerstitium (tubular atrophy and interstitial inflammation and fibrosis) (Fig 8.4).

Main consequences of chronic kidney disease

The manifestations of CKD are protean, and affect every organ system of the body (Fig. 8.5). They arise because the kidneys fail to perform their usual excretory, regulatory, metabolic and biosynthetic functions. The current patient developed many of these problems. See 8.1: 2.

The uraemic syndrome refers to the composite clinical picture arising from concurrent appearance of many of these manifestations, but in particular those arising from the failure to excrete nitrogenous compounds

Fig. 8.3 Photomicrograph illustrating features of diabetic nephropathy. Note (a) the thickening of glomerular capillary walls, (b) nodule formation, (c) hyaline thickening of the arteriolar wall, and (d) interstitial scarring.

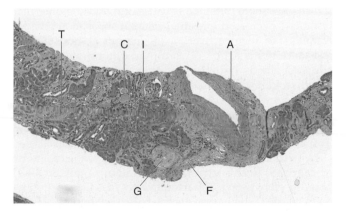

Fig. 8.4 Photomicrograph illustrating an end-stage kidney with glomerulosclerosis (G), interstitial inflammation (I) and fibrosis (F), atrophic and dilated tubules (T) containing casts (C) and thickened arteries (A).

(such as urea) and other 'uraemic toxins', many of which remain poorly defined. In general, there is a poor correlation between the systemic concentration of most of these substances and uraemic symptomatology. In particular, anorexia, nausea and vomiting are common uraemic symptoms, but drowsiness, lethargy, pruritus (itch), neuropathy and pericarditis can be seen when the condition is advanced.

It is sometimes difficult to differentiate symptoms of the primary disease (in this case diabetes mellitus) from those of kidney failure, either because the symptoms are non-specific or because both diseases cause similar organ damage. For example, both diabetes and renal failure can be complicated by myocardial and peripheral ischaemia, and by peripheral neuropathy. Shared symptoms may thus arise earlier in the course of diabetic CKD than would be the case with other primary diseases.

Hypertension occurs mainly because of failure to excrete salt and water adequately. The resulting expansion in extracellular fluid volume triggers release of a natriuretic hormone from the central nervous system as a compensatory measure, but this also acts as a peripheral vasoconstrictor. Other contributing mechanisms may include increased renin (and therefore angiotensin) production by the scarred and ischaemic kidney, and reduced renal production of vasodepressor hormones (see Chapter 10). Peripheral oedema commonly develops and the patient may have all the features of congestive cardiac failure. While net retention of salt and water is

---

Case 8.1 — Diabetic nephropathy and CKD: 2

Disease progression

Over the next few years Raylene's kidney impairment continued to worsen slowly. She became progressively lethargic, due mainly to the development of anaemia. Her blood pressure became more difficult to control, as did her oedema. She developed mild pain in the long bones of her lower limbs, as well as generalized pruritus. On one occasion she presented with sudden shortness of breath, thought to be because of myocardial ischaemia. Her feet became numb, and a 2 cm ulcer developed on the plantar surface of her right hallux (big toe).

The progressive decline of kidney function invites the following questions:

1. Why does this happen?
2. Can anything be done to prevent it?

The patient's symptoms were thought to be caused by complications of uraemia, affecting her bone marrow, bones, skin, central and peripheral blood vessels and peripheral nerves. In the next section, complications and consequences of CKD will be discussed.

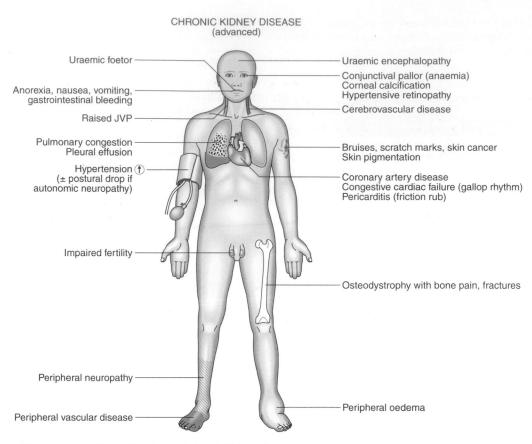

CHRONIC KIDNEY DISEASE
(advanced)

Uraemic foetor

Anorexia, nausea, vomiting,
gastrointestinal bleeding

Raised JVP

Pulmonary congestion
Pleural effusion

Hypertension (↑)
(± postural drop if
autonomic neuropathy)

Impaired fertility

Peripheral neuropathy

Peripheral vascular disease

Uraemic encephalopathy
Conjunctival pallor (anaemia)
Corneal calcification
Hypertensive retinopathy
Cerebrovascular disease

Bruises, scratch marks, skin cancer
Skin pigmentation

Coronary artery disease
Congestive cardiac failure (gallop rhythm)
Pericarditis (friction rub)

Osteodystrophy with bone pain, fractures

Peripheral oedema

Fig. 8.5 Characteristic signs in a patient with advanced chronic kidney disease.

usual, the capacity of the kidney to concentrate the urine and maximally reabsorb sodium is also impaired so, paradoxically, the patient is at risk of volume depletion in the face of restricted intake of salt and water. Overall, the range of homeostatic responses to changes in salt and water intake is greatly narrowed in chronic kidney disease.

Interesting facts

Nocturia is one of the earliest symptoms of CKD, first occurring when GFR is less than half normal. When this symptom has been present for some time prior to presentation, it is useful for differentiating chronic from acute kidney disease. It occurs because loss of concentrating ability with reduced GFR means that obligate excretion of urinary solutes requires greater volumes of urine, particularly at night when urine concentration is normally maximal.

Because of efficient renal adaptive mechanisms, hyperkalaemia (arising from a failure to excrete potassium) is usually a late manifestation of kidney failure. The renal adaptation consists of enhanced potassium secretion in the distal tubule. Failure to excrete acid leads to a generally mild metabolic acidosis, which contributes to renal osteodystrophy and malnutrition.

Renal osteodystrophy refers to the bone disease which occurs with CKD. It arises because of a complex interplay between calcium, phosphate, acidosis, parathyroid hormone and vitamin D (Fig. 8.6). The principal hormones involved in renal osteodystrophy are parathyroid hormone and activated vitamin D (calcitriol). The simplified physiology of both is summarized in Table 8.4. Reduction in serum ionized calcium concentration plays a central role. This occurs because of precipitation with elevated serum phosphate (retained because of reduced glomerular filtration), decreased intestinal calcium absorption because of failure of renal activation of vitamin D, and skeletal resistance to the action of parathyroid hormone. The parathyroid glands hypertrophy and secrete high levels of parathyroid hormone (secondary hyperparathyroidism) in response to the falling serum calcium. Activation of vitamin D (cholecalciferol) normally occurs by two hydroxylation steps, the first in the liver (25-hydroxylation) to form 25-hydroxycholecalciferol, and the second in the kidney (1-hydroxylation) to form 1,25-dihydroxycholecalciferol, or calcitriol. Renal activation of vitamin D fails in CKD because of hyperphosphataemia and loss of functioning renal tissue, which prevents 1-hydroxylation of 25-OH vitamin D. The bone disease comprises a variable mix of hyperparathyroidism (causing **osteitis fibrosa cystica**), **osteomalacia** and **osteoporosis**. In addition, hyperphosphataemia leads to **metastatic calcification** in most organs,

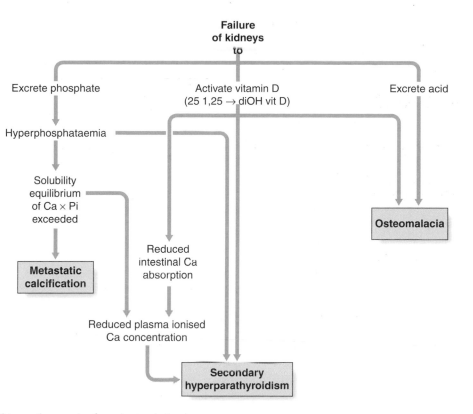

Fig. 8.6 Schema describing pathogenesis of renal osteodystrophy.

including the skin (where it can cause pruritus), blood vessels, heart and joints.

Atheromatous occlusive vascular disease can impair circulation to all organs, in particular to the heart, brain and lower limbs. Almost half the patients with ESKD die from cardiovascular events. Atheroma arises owing to multiple factors in patients with kidney failure, including hypertension, dyslipidaemia and metastatic calcification, sometimes aggravated by cigarette smoking.

Interesting facts

Over a 5-year period, 20–25% of patients with stage 2 or 3 CKD die, usually from cardiovascular disease, whereas only 2% reach end-stage kidney disease (ESKD). The situation is similar for stage 4 CKD, where 45–50% die in 5 years, yet only 20% progress to ESKD.

A common early symptom in CKD is lethargy, caused mainly by normochromic normocytic anaemia resulting from failure of renal erythropoietin production. Erythropoietin (or epoetin) is secreted predominantly as a glycoprotein of 165 amino acids by fibroblast-like interstitial cells in the kidney, in response to anaemia and hypoxia. Its synthesis falls as renal scarring progresses, with a consequential fall in red cell mass as its stimulatory effect on the bone marrow is lost. The reduced capacity of the blood to carry oxygen because of deficiency of erythropoietin is a major cause of morbidity in patients with

CKD, and management of this problem has been revolutionized by the availability of synthetic erythropoietin as replacement therapy. In contrast, white blood cells and platelets are normal in number, but their impaired function contributes to a predisposition to infection and a bleeding tendency, respectively.

There are many other manifestations of CKD, some common and some rare. These are summarized in Tables 8.5 and 8.6 and illustrated in Fig. 8.5.

Progression of chronic kidney disease

As illustrated by the current case, once kidney impairment has become severe enough the disease tends to progress through the various stages outlined in Table 8.2 to end-stage. This occurs even when the primary disease causing kidney impairment has become inactive. However, if the primary disease becomes quiescent (either through natural or treatment-induced reparative processes) before kidney functional impairment and scarring have become critically severe, then CKD may not be progressive.

The factors causing progression of CKD are not entirely clear, but a number of implicated factors are listed in Box 8.2. Two mechanisms receiving considerable attention over the past two decades are systemic and intraglomerular hypertension, and proteinuria.

Increased glomerular hydrostatic pressure has been observed directly in several experimental models of CKD,

Table 8.4 Simplified physiology of parathyroid hormone and calcitriol production and action

Parathyroid hormone	Calcitriol (activated vitamin D)
Production	**Activation**
Polypeptide with 84 amino acids secreted by parathyroid chief cells	Sterol activated by hydroxylase in kidney
(+) by low plasma ionized Ca^{2+} and high plasma P_i	(+) by parathyroid hormone
(−) by high plasma ionized Ca^{2+} and calcitriol	(−) by high plasma P_i concentration
Action	**Action**
Kidney $\uparrow R_{Ca}^{2+}$, $\downarrow R_{Pi}$	$\uparrow R_{Ca}^{2+}$, $\uparrow R_{Pi}$
(+) 1α hydroxylase	
Bone $\uparrow$ turnover (osteoblastic formation and osteoclastic resorption)	$\uparrow$ Bone mineralization
Parathyroids –	(−) Parathyroid hormone release
Gut –	$\uparrow Ca^{2+}$ and P_i absorption

R, tubular reabsorption; (+) stimulates or stimulated; (−), inhibits or inhibited; P_i, inorganic phosphate.

Table 8.5 Main consequences of CKD

Mechanism	Example	Consequence
Decreased excretion	Uraemic toxins, including nitrogenous wastes	Uraemic syndrome
	Salt and water	Volume overload, hypertension
	Phosphate	Hyperparathyroidism, metastatic calcification
	Acid	Metabolic acidosis
	Potassium	Hyperkalaemia
Decreased biosynthesis	Erythropoietin	Anaemia
	Activation of vitamin D	Osteomalacia, hyperparathyroidism
Altered metabolism	Dyslipidaemia	Atherogenesis
	Sex hormones	Abnormal reproductive function

Table 8.6 Organ system involvement in CKD

System	Main pathogenetic factors	Main consequences
Cardiovascular	Atheroma	Occlusive vascular disease
	Salt and water retention	Hypertension, 'congestive cardiac failure'
Bone	Secondary hyperparathyroidism	Pain, rarely fracture
	Osteomalacia	
	Osteoporosis	
Neuromuscular	'Uraemic toxins'	Sensorimotor peripheral neuropathy
		Autonomic neuropathy
		Encephalopathy
Blood	Erythropoietin deficiency	Anaemia
	'Uraemic toxins'	Impaired white cell and platelet function
Skin	Metastatic calcification	Pruritus
	Sun exposure	Skin cancer
	Anaemia and 'uraemic toxins'	Sallow complexion
Reproductive	Abnormal regulation of sex hormones	Reduced libido, impaired fertility
Gastrointestinal	'Uraemic toxins'	Anorexia, nausea, vomiting, malnutrition
Serosal	'Uraemic toxins'	Pericarditis

Box 8.2 Factors causing progression of CKD

Renal	Systemic
Continuing activity of primary disease	Systemic hypertension
Intraglomerular hypertension	Smoking
Proteinuria	Obesity
Nephrocalcinosis (dystrophic and metastatic)	Dyslipidaemia
Imbalance between renal energy demands and supply	Excess dietary protein

Box 8.3 Causes of acute deterioration of kidney function in patients with CKD

Recrudescence of primary disease
Complication of primary disease
Accelerated hypertension
Volume depletion
Cardiac failure
Sepsis
Nephrotoxins (radiocontrast, drugs*)
Renal artery occlusion
Urinary tract obstruction
Dietary protein load

*Including especially non-steroidal anti-inflammatory drugs and, in some situations, angiotensin-converting enzyme inhibitors and angiotensin receptor blockers (see Chapter 14).

and inferred in some forms of human CKD such as diabetic nephropathy. The resultant haemodynamic injury ('hyperfiltration') has been proposed to lead to progressive glomerular scarring.

Proteinuria is not merely a manifestation of CKD, but also an important factor leading to progressive kidney scarring. It is thought that reabsorbed protein causes tubular cell damage, and also leads to tubular cell production of cytokines which incite an inflammatory and fibrogenic response in the surrounding interstitium. The net effect of these and other factors is progressive scarring of glomeruli and tubulointerstitial areas of the kidney.

This non-specific progression of CKD needs to be distinguished from separate events which may lead to superimposed acute kidney injury; that is, acute-on-chronic kidney disease (Box 8.3). For example, falls in extracellular fluid volume or blood pressure are commonly associated with an acute deterioration of GFR in a patient with otherwise stable CKD. When the abnormality can be corrected in a timely fashion, GFR should return to baseline. However, when the abnormality is sustained or cannot be corrected (for example, with acute renal artery occlusion in a patient with renal artery stenosis), then GFR may not improve.

Case 8.1 Diabetic nephropathy and CKD: 3

End-stage disease

Raylene's kidney failure continued to deteriorate and she was started on several different drugs to control blood pressure, fluid retention, hyperphosphataemia and acidosis. Her diet was adjusted to restrict salt, potassium, protein and fluid intake.

Three years after her presentation with CKD she was started on haemodialysis and placed on the waiting list to receive a cadaveric renal transplant.

Principles of treatment

After establishing the aetiology and severity of CKD, management is directed towards detection and treatment of factors that may cause superimposed acute kidney injury or non-specific progression, and of complications of CKD (Box 8.4). Of particular importance is the control of systemic hypertension and reduction of proteinuria, for the reasons explained above. The various fluid and electrolyte and metabolic disturbances of CKD may respond well to dietary manipulation and drugs. For example, restriction of excessive dietary protein, salt, potassium, phosphate, water and saturated fats may all be necessary at some stage. Hyperphosphataemia, metabolic acidosis and sodium retention may be treated with phosphate binders (such as oral calcium carbonate), sodium bicarbonate supplements, and loop diuretics, respectively. Erythropoietin (by injection) and calcitriol may be given to replace deficiencies of those hormones. Smoking has been shown unequivocally to worsen atheromatous disease as well as promote progression of renal disease, and should be stringently avoided, especially in diabetic patients.

In the majority of patients, CKD follows a predictable course. Thus, continuing surveillance for treatable complications and a planned transition to ESKD therapy (dialysis and transplantation) is possible and desirable.

Box 8.4 Principles of treatment of patients with CKD

Differentiate from acute kidney injury (Table 8.1)
Establish aetiology (Table 8.3)
Establish severity (Table 8.2)
Seek and treat reversible factors (Box 8.3)
Seek and treat complications (Table 8.6)
Lifestyle changes (diet, exercise, cease smoking, avoid polypharmacy)
Seek and treat factors causing progression (Box 8.2)
Planned transition to dialysis and transplantation (Chapter 9)

END-STAGE KIDNEY DISEASE AND REPLACEMENT OF RENAL FUNCTION

Chapter objectives

After studying this chapter you should be able to understand:

1. What kidney functions can be replaced by dialysis and transplantation.

2. The principles and modes of dialysis.

3. How to prepare a patient for chronic dialysis.

4. The outcomes and complications of chronic dialysis.

5. The differences between dialysis for acute versus end-stage kidney disease.

6. Modes of transplantation.

7. How to prepare a patient for transplantation.

8. Outcomes and complications of transplantation.

9. Conservative management of end-stage kidney disease.

Introduction

Renal replacement therapy refers to treatment of a patient with advanced loss of renal function using dialysis and kidney transplantation. Dialysis may be required to replace kidney function temporarily in a patient with acute kidney injury (AKI), or long term in a patient with end-stage kidney disease (ESKD). Kidney transplantation may be used to replace kidney function in a patient with end-stage kidney disease, but is not used as treatment of acute kidney injury.

This chapter gives an overview of these forms of treatment based on consideration of two typical case histories.

Interesting facts

Currently there are at least two million people with ESKD world-wide and more than 300 million people with early vascular disease and kidney dysfunction who are at risk of cardiovascular disease and ESKD.

Case 9.1 Dialysis for end-stage kidney disease: 1

Roland Walkum is a 68-year-old man with chronic kidney disease due to chronic glomerulonephritis. His renal function slowly deteriorated over 5 years until his GFR fell to about 10 mL per minute and he developed symptoms of uraemia and fluid overload, including nausea and dyspnoea. He was otherwise a healthy man who did not wish to die from his kidney disease. When the options were explained to him, he opted to commence treatment with peritoneal dialysis as it best suited his lifestyle. A peritoneal dialysis catheter was placed and he was trained to perform continuous ambulatory peritoneal dialysis at home. After dialysis was commenced, he was able to stop or reduce the dose of several medications that he had been taking to treat and prevent the complications of chronic kidney disease. Apart from several episodes of peritonitis and exit site infection, he tolerated peritoneal dialysis very well. After 4 years on peritoneal dialysis he slowly developed progressive oedema which was unresponsive to changes in his dialysis regimen. An arteriovenous fistula was created in his left forearm, and he was switched to haemodialysis.

Several issues arise from this case history:

1. What are the different modes of dialysis delivery, and what factors govern the choice?
2. How should a patient be prepared for chronic dialysis?
3. What are the long–term complications and outcomes of dialysis?

Replacement of kidney function

Once chronic kidney disease has progressed to stage 5 (GFR $< 15\,mL/min/1.73\,m^2$), death from renal failure will ensue in a relatively short timeframe unless some form of replacement of kidney function is provided.

Successful kidney transplantation can replace up to half of total normal kidney function since a single kidney is transplanted. Potentially this is sufficient to adequately replace all functions of the normal kidney. In contrast, dialysis is able to replace only some of the functions performed by a normal kidney. It has the potential to replace most of the kidney's role in regulating fluid and electrolyte balance and to remove low molecular weight solutes, but is only partially effective at regulating calcium and phosphate balance, controlling blood pressure, and removing larger solutes, and is unable to replace any of the hormonal and synthetic functions of the normal kidney (see Box 9.1). As a consequence, supplementary dietary and drug treatment is required in nearly all patients on dialysis (see Table 9.1).

Most of these supplementary therapies are required in progressively higher doses in patients with CKD as kidney function deteriorates. Once the patient commences dialysis, the need for supplemental therapy may disappear (e.g. sodium bicarbonate), diminish (e.g. some dietary restrictions, phosphate binders and antihypertensives) or continue (e.g. erythropoietin, calcitriol).

Box 9.1 Replacement of kidney function by dialysis

Complete*	Partial**	Nil
Regulation of ECFV	Control of blood pressure	Metabolism of filtered proteins
Regulation of osmolality	Excretion of middle molecular range solutes	Synthesis of erythropoietin
Regulation of acid–base balance	Excretion of 'uraemic toxins'	Synthesis of renin–angiotensin
Regulation of potassium balance	Regulation of calcium and phosphate balance	Synthesis of their other local hormones
Excretion of low molecular weight solutes		Activation of 250 H vitamin D

*Potentially these functions can be completely replaced by optimal dialysis, but may require some supplementary therapy.
**Replacement of these functions usually requires additional drug therapy.
ECFV = extracellular fluid volume.

These changes depend on the extent to which dialysis can replace individual kidney functions (see Box 9.1).

Principles and modes of dialysis

Dialysis literally means the separation of a substance across a membrane. Clinically, it is used to refer to any process by which solutes (including drugs and toxins) are removed from the body fluids through an artificial intervention, using either an external circuit through which the blood is passed (haemodialysis) or the lining of the peritoneal cavity (peritoneal dialysis).

Haemodialysis

Interesting facts

Haemodialysis was first used to save human life during World War II by a Dutch physician, Willem Kolff. From the 1960s haemodialysis became more widely available due to the development of artificial shunts (by Belding Scribner) and arteriovenous fistulas (by Brescia and Cimino).

In haemodialysis, the patient's blood flows through an artificial kidney countercurrent to, and separated by a semipermeable membrane from, dialysis fluid (see Fig. 9.1).

Table 9.1 Supplementary therapy

Function*	Supplementary therapy
Regulation of ECFV	Appropriate sodium and water intake; loop diuretic if passing urine
Regulation of osmolality	Appropriate water intake
Regulation of potassium balance	Dietary K restriction with HD, occasional use of K-binding resin (resonium); sometimes dietary K supplementation with PD
Regulation of calcium/ phosphate balance	Phosphate binders, calcitriol, calcimimetic drug
Regulation of magnesium	Avoid excessive magnesium intake
Synthesis of erythropoietin	Erythropoietin or its analoques
Synthesis of renin– angiotensin	Sometimes ACEi or ARB
Activation of 25OH vitamin D	Calcitriol

*For other normal kidney functions (listed in Box 9.1) supplemental therapy is either unnecessary or not available. ECFV = extracellular fluid volume, ACEi = angiotensin converting enzyme inhibitor, ARB = angiotensin receptor blocker.

Solute removal from the body across the dialysis membrane occurs by diffusion down the solute's concentration gradient (best for low molecular weight solutes, less than 500 daltons) or by convection in which solutes are dragged along with water (best for larger molecules, greater than 500 daltons). The amount of fluid and solutes removed can be varied by regulating the flows of blood and dialysate and the pressures in the blood and dialysate compartments, and by using dialysis membranes with different permeabilities.

Haemodialysis for patients with ESKD may be delivered in hospital, in a satellite unit specialising in dialysis or at home. In most patients, dialysis is delivered for four to five hours three times a week. This can replace approximately 10% of glomerular filtration rate (GFR). By increasing the hours of dialysis and to a lesser extent blood flow rates, dialysis delivery can be increased substantially. Some patients with very long dialysis hours (e.g. overnight dialysis, most nights per week) can achieve such good replacement of kidney function that the need for supplemental therapy (e.g. phosphate binders, antihypertensives, erythropoietin) can be obviated or greatly reduced.

Dialysis for patients with acute kidney injury (AKI) is usually delivered in intensive care or high dependency units by continuous or extended hour therapy.

Peritoneal dialysis

Alternatively peritoneal dialysis can be used for patients with ESKD. In this situation the peritoneal membrane, the endothelium of peritoneal blood vessels and the supporting tissue between the two, act jointly as the semipermeable membrane. Except in situations where haemodialysis is not available, peritoneal dialysis is rarely used for treatment of patients with AKI (see Box 9.2). Peritoneal dialysis may be administered by machine, usually overnight (automated peritoneal dialysis), or by manual exchanges during the day and night (continuous ambulatory peritoneal dialysis, or CAPD).

Table 9.2 gives some data for the population of patients undergoing chronic dialysis in Australia in 2006.

Preparing a patient for chronic dialysis

The best outcomes in dialysis can be achieved if the patient has a planned transition from treatment of progressive chronic kidney disease (CKD) to dialysis. Patients who need to start dialysis urgently often run into problems with dialysis access, as well as complications of ESKD such as fluid overload.

During stage 4 CKD (GFR 15–30 mL per minute/ $1.73\,m^2$) patients should receive education about ESKD therapy so they can make an informed decision about choice of dialysis modality. In the absence of medical and psychological contraindications, patient choice is the

Fig. 9.1 Principles of haemodialysis.

Box 9.2 Modes of dialysis delivery

For AKI	For ESKD
Intermittent haemodialysis	Haemodialysis – home, satellite or hospital
Continuous venovenous haemodialysis (CVVHD)	Automated peritoneal dialysis (APD)
Slow low efficiency daily dialysis (SLEDD)	Continuous ambulatory peritoneal dialysis (CAPD)
Acute peritoneal dialysis (rarely)	

AKI = acute kidney injury; ESKD = end-stage kidney disease.

Box 9.3 Relative medical contraindications to home

Peritoneal dialysis	Home haemodialysis
Previous abdominal surgery with adhesions	Vasculature unsuitable for AV fistula
Unrepaired abdominal herniae	Severe cardiovascular disease
Bowel diseases (e.g. diverticulitis)	Other severe medical conditions
Serious lung disease	
Abdominal obesity	

Table 9.2	Renal replacement therapy in Australia, 2006	
Patients on dialysis		9200
New patients (in 2006)		1700
PD	APD	10%
	CAPD	10%
HD	Hospital	25%
	Home	10%
	Satellite	45%

most important determinant of initial mode of therapy. The patient's social and psychological wellbeing, suitability for home dialysis and suitability for PD versus HD needs to be assessed (see Box 9.3). During this phase

it is necessary to correct reversible factors that preclude the dialysis modality chosen by the patient. The patient needs to be assessed for presence of infectious diseases (hepatitis B & C, HIV, MRSA, VRE) and, if they have no antibodies to hepatitis B, receive vaccination against hepatitis B. Their potential for receiving a kidney transplant also needs to be assessed.

In addition to patient preference, the modality of dialysis is determined by the presence or not of various medical, psychological and social factors. For example, in patients with previous major abdominal surgery with peritoneal adhesions, unrepaired herniae, bowel conditions such as diverticulitis and severe respiratory insufficiency, peritoneal dialysis may not be possible. In patients with blood vessels unsuitable for permanent vascular access and some medical comorbidities such as

Box 9.4 When to initiate dialysis

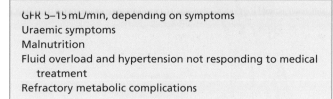

GFR 5–15 mL/min, depending on symptoms
Uraemic symptoms
Malnutrition
Fluid overload and hypertension not responding to medical
   treatment
Refractory metabolic complications

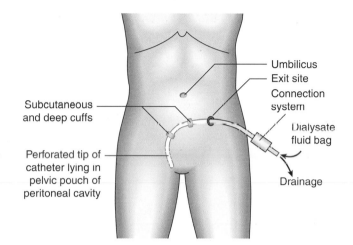

Fig. 9.2 Peritoneal dialysis catheter.

severe cardiovascular disease, haemodialysis may not be possible. In addition, peritoneal dialysis is unable to deliver as much solute clearance as haemodialysis and may be less suitable for large patients with minimal or no remaining native kidney function.

Dialysis should be initiated before the patient has developed severe symptoms of kidney failure. Whereas dialysis is usually commenced when the patient's GFR has fallen to between 5 and 15 mL per minute, more important determinants of when to start dialysis than GFR *per se* are uraemic symptoms, worsening nutrition, poor blood pressure and fluid control and refractory metabolic complications of kidney failure (see Box 9.4).

Interesting facts

Residual kidney function continues to deteriorate once a patient commences dialysis, more quickly with HD than PD. Once residual kidney function is lost, some patients on PD need to transfer to HD.

Dialysis access

For peritoneal dialysis, a catheter is placed in the peritoneal cavity (see Fig. 9.2). The catheter usually exits the peritoneal cavity in the midline below the umbilicus, courses along a subcutaneous tunnel and exits the abdominal wall laterally. To reduce the risk of leakage of peritoneal fluid from the exit site, it is advisable for the catheter to be in place for two to four weeks prior to use.

Permanent haemodialysis access is best achieved using an arteriovenous (AV) fistula in which an artery (frequently radial artery) is anastomosed end-to-side or side-to-side to a vein (cephalic vein in the case of radial artery) (see Fig. 9.3). The vein becomes 'arterialized' due to the increased pressure and flow of blood through it, and is suitable for recurrent cannulation after about six weeks. Alternatively an AV graft may be constructed by the use of a synthetic conduit material or a harvested (e.g. saphenous) vein. In patients with poor peripheral blood vessels, especially when immediate access is required, it may be necessary to use a synthetic venous catheter, usually placed in the internal jugular vein and preferably with a subcutaneous tunnel to reduce the risk of catheter infection (see Fig. 9.4).

Outcomes and complications of chronic dialysis

Morbidity in chronic dialysis patients arises from complications of the dialysis procedure itself, from continuing inadequately controlled consequences of kidney failure, or from accompanying medical conditions. The most frequent complications of peritoneal dialysis include infection (peritonitis, exit site infection, tunnel infection) or gradual failure of the peritoneal membrane to effectively transport solutes and water.

Complications of haemodialysis include infection, stenosis and thrombosis of the vascular access, problems during the haemodialysis procedure itself (e.g. hypotension) or problems occurring between treatments (usually due to excessive intake of water and solutes) (see Box 9.5). Intercurrent cardiovascular disease is common in patients with ESKD and a frequent cause of morbidity and mortality. The most common causes of death amongst dialysis patients are cardiac events (myocardial infarction and sudden death) and withdrawal from dialysis for various reasons (see Table 9.3).

Dialysis for acute kidney injury

Acute kidney injury (AKI, also known as acute renal failure) is common amongst hospitalized patients, particularly patients with multi-organ failure and patients with cardiac disease in intensive care and high dependency units. If AKI is severe enough dialysis may be necessary until kidney function recovers. As these patients are frequently quite unwell, dialysis is often commenced at higher levels of GFR and with higher doses of dialysis than for patients with ESKD. Although complications of the dialysis procedure are relatively common (infection, cardiovascular instability), patient outcome is largely determined by the underlying disease. Dialysis partially replaces kidney function but in general does not affect

Fig. 9.3 (A) Arteriovenous fistula and (B) graft for haemodialysis.

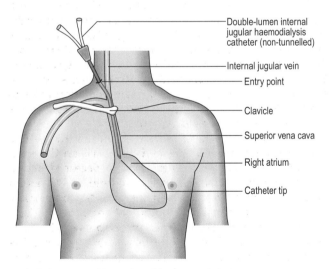

Fig. 9.4 Internal jugular catheter for haemodialysis.

Box 9.5 Common complications of chronic dialysis

Peritoneal dialysis (PD)
Infection – catheter exit site tunnel, peritonitis
Poor drainage of or leaking dialysate

Haemodialysis (HD)
Vascular access – infection, thrombosis, stenosis
Accidents during dialysis – blood loss, clotting of artificial kidney (dialyser)
Haemodynamic instability during dialysis

PD & HD
Insufficient dialysis
Inadequate nutrition
Fluid overload
Accelerated atherogenesis

the vunderlying disease or cause of kidney failure, nor does it hasten the recovery of kidney function. Patients with AKI may require dialysis for periods ranging from a few days to several weeks.

Peritoneal dialysis is now used infrequently for AKI, except in areas where availability of haemodialysis is limited. When used immediately, as is usually required for AKI, peritoneal dialysis catheters are subject to the leakage of dialysate (and therefore risk of infection).

In a stable patient with AKI, haemodialysis may be delivered intermittently, as it is for patients with ESKD.

However, many patients with AKI are quite unwell and are better dialysed with a slow continuous form of therapy which is characterized by greater cardiovascular stability. Most commonly patients are dialysed continuously via catheters placed in large veins (continuous venovenous haemodialysis). As the blood is not arterial, an external pump is required to pump blood through the artificial kidney. Usually dialysis is combined with filtration (convection) to allow optimal clearance of solutes,

Table 9.3 Causes of death in ESKD patients

	Dialysis	Transplant
Cardiac	35%	30%
Withdrawal from treatment	35%	5%
Infection	10%	15%
Vascular	10%	15%
Malignancy	5%	30%
Miscellaneous	5%	5%

so-called haemodiafiltration. There is an increasing trend to use a dialysis treatment that combines the advantages of intermittent haemodialysis and CVVHD, so-called slow low efficiency daily dialysis (SLEDD). Adequate removal of solutes and water can be achieved by dialysis for eight to twelve hours per day, allowing time for patients to attend investigations and receive other treatments while not on dialysis. In addition to removing the usual toxins of kidney failure, dialysis may also remove inflammatory mediators involved in the patient's multiorgan failure.

Case 9.2

Transplantation for end-stage kidney disease: 1

Cindy Lopez is a 50-year-old female with polycystic kidney disease. Her disease has been progressing slowly towards end-stage, and her latest GFR was 20 mL/min/1.73 m². Apart from occasional macroscopic haematuria and kidney pain, she was asymptomatic. Her blood pressure, fluids and electrolytes were all well controlled by diet and medications. Cindy was not keen to have dialysis because her mother, who also had polycystic kidney disease, had died 15 years ago while on dialysis. Cindy has three brothers, two of whom are well with no kidney disease. Cindy is blood group A, as is one of her brothers; her other brother is blood group O. Cindy would like to receive a transplant from one of her brothers and not have dialysis.

This case raises the following questions:

1. Can she receive a kidney transplant without dialysis?
2. Would it be better for her to wait to receive a transplant from the deceased donor waiting list?
3. What are the likely outcomes of her transplantation?

Principles and modes of transplantation

Renal transplantation is a well-established form of treatment for end-stage kidney disease, available in most parts of the developed world and increasingly in some developing countries. Its successful delivery depends on access to high standards of care from a team involving transplant surgeons, nephrologists, immunologists, infectious diseases experts and other personnel. The account given here introduces only some principles of the procedure and its consequences.

Interesting facts

The first functioning human allograft was placed in 1946. However it wasn't until immunosuppressive therapy became available in the 1960s that transplantation became a routine clinical reality.

Modes of transplantation

Kidney transplants may be obtained from a living donor or from a deceased donor. Living donors are either related by blood (e.g. parents, siblings) or are emotionally linked (e.g. spouse, close friend). Very occasionally 'altruistic' donation occurs from an unrelated living donor, but transplantation for profit (so called 'organ trafficking') is illegal. Living related donation has the potential advantage of greater histocompatibility and therefore potentially better outcomes, but the results of spousal donation are almost as good. Until recently transplantation did not occur across ABO blood group incompatibilities. However, excellent long-term results are now being achieved with ABO incompatible transplantation, using plasma exchange and immunosuppression to remove the recipient's anti-donor blood group antibodies prior to transplantation. Living donation can occur either before dialysis, or when a patient is already on dialysis. Transplantation prior to dialysis (so called 'pre-emptive' transplantation) has the obvious advantage of avoidance of dialysis.

If there are no potential living donors then the patient needs to commence dialysis and be placed on the waiting list to receive a transplant from a deceased donor. Deceased donor transplantation requires ABO blood group compatibility and histocompatibility. Preference is given to donor–recipient pairs that share major histocompatibility antigens, and also to recipients who have been on the transplant waiting list for long periods. The number of patients awaiting transplantation is much greater than the number of available transplants and so the number of patients on the transplant waiting list and the mean waiting time prior to transplantation are increasing steadily in most western countries.

Usually one kidney is transplanted, extraperitoneally in the iliac fossa (Fig. 9.5). For a small number of patients with diabetes and kidney disease, pancreas and kidney are transplanted at the same time.

Preparing a patient for transplantation

Factors that determine whether a patient is deemed fit enough to receive a kidney transplant include the

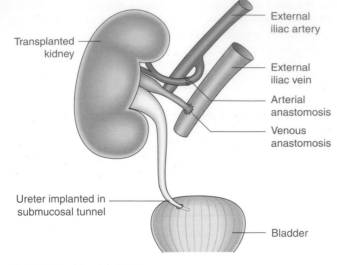

Fig. 9.5 Renal transplantation.

operative risk, the risk of loss of the transplant due to technical and immunological reasons, and the risks associated with immunosuppression. The cardiovascular health of the patient is an important determinant of the safety of the anaesthetic and surgery, and long-term outcome. Age *per se* is not important but in patients over age 60 (or in diabetics of more than 50 years) it is important to exclude significant cardiovascular disease. The risks of transplant loss relate to local factors (such as diseased iliac blood vessels, bladder abnormalities), recurrent disease in the transplant (such as can occur with focal sclerosing and mesangial IgA glomerulonephritis) and heightened risk of rejection (as in a patient who is sensitized against donor antigens or has previously rejected a transplant). In patients with ongoing infection (including chronic hepatitis, HIV, latent tuberculosis) or heightened cancer risk, the need for immunosuppressive therapy to prevent transplant rejection may carry too great a risk of infection or malignancy.

If a patient is deemed fit for transplantation then they submit a blood sample monthly to assess the development of immune responses which would increase the risk of transplant rejection. As the waiting time for a kidney from a deceased donor is frequently quite prolonged, it is important that the patient's various risk factors are reassessed at regular intervals.

In patients who receive a living donor transplant, the processes of recipient assessment are similar. In addition, the likelihood of immunological response of the recipient to the donated kidney is more readily determined than with a deceased donor transplant.

In considering whether an individual is fit to donate a kidney, a prime consideration is whether the donation would increase the risk of deterioration in the remaining kidney. In a patient with a personal or family history of diabetes, hypertension or other diseases which may affect kidney function, the risk to the potential donor may not be acceptable. Potential donors need to have a total GFR

of greater than $80\,mL/min/1.73\,m^2$ (so that after donation they are left with a GFR of at least half this amount) and no evidence of structural disease of the kidneys, urinary tract and renal blood vessels.

In the case of deceased donor transplantation, patients will receive only a few hours warning before the transplantation must proceed. In addition to the considerations above, they must have no acute health concerns, such as active infection. In the case of live donor transplantation prior to dialysis the donation should occur prior to the development of significant symptoms of ESKD, usually when the GFR is about or greater than $10–15\,mL/min/1.73\,m^2$.

Outcomes and complications of transplantation

With modern immunosuppression, transplant and recipient outcomes have improved markedly over the last couple of decades. The one and five year survival for a deceased donor transplant in Australia is currently 90 and 80% respectively, and patient survival is 95 and 90%. The outcomes after living donation are even better. The transplant may rarely be lost early due to surgical problems or acute rejection. Acute rejection now occurs in less than a third of patients during the first 12 months and accounts for less than 15% of grafts lost during that period. Patients at increased risk of acute rejection include those with high percentage of antibodies against common histocompatibility antigens, donor-specific antibodies and prior transplant loss from acute rejection. Transplants may be lost in the long term because of chronic rejection, nephrotoxicity of immunosuppressive drugs (calcineurin inhibitors), recurrence of the disease which caused ESKD (such as glomerulonephritis or diabetes) or patient death with a functioning transplant. Amongst the immunosuppressive agents, calcineurin inhibitors (such as cyclosporin and tacrolimus) can lead to progressive loss of graft function. So called 'chronic allograft nephropathy' is multifactoral, and is due to chronic immunological processes, calcineurin nephrotoxicity and other factors.

Recipients of a kidney transplant remain on immunosuppressive medications for life, since even late withdrawal will usually result in loss of the transplant by rejection. Commonly used immunosuppressive agents are listed in Table 9.4. The majority of patients receive three or four different agents initially, falling to one to three agents in lower doses after a year or so. Initial therapy frequently includes biological agents (anti-IL2 antibody, or lymphocyte-depleting agents for those at high risk of transplant rejection). The reduction in immunosuppressive therapy over time is individualized, based on the patient's record of (or potential for) adverse events. Patient non-adherence to therapy is a major concern.

Immunosuppressive therapy increases the risk of infection, and also malignancies. In 2006 malignancy accounted for more than 30% of transplant patient mortality in Australia, while cardiac disease caused 30% and

Table 9.4 Immunosuppressive agents used to prevent kidney transplant rejection, and their common side effects

Drug class/example	Common side effects
Corticosteroids	
Prednisolone	Hypertension, osteopenia, dyslipidaemia, diabetes
Calcineurin inhibitors	
Cyclosporine	Nephrotoxicity, hypertension
Tacrolimus	Diabetes, hypertension, nephrotoxicity
mTOR inhibitors	
Sirolimus, everolimus	Poor wound healing, proteinuria, dyslipidaemia
Antiproliferative agents	
Azathioprine	Myelosuppression
Mycophenolate	Gastrointestinal disturbances, myelosuppression

mTOR, mammalian target of rapamycin (sirolimus).

infection 15% of deaths (see Table 9.3). During the first three to six months patients receive agents to prevent the risk of bacterial infection (pneumocystis pneumonia and urinary tract infection), fungal infection (usually oral) and viral infection (CMV etc). Patients may have ongoing renal osteodystrophy and osteoporosis (from steroid therapy) which requires treatment with various agents such as bisphosphonates and vitamin D. Many patients also require chronic treatment for hypertension. Finally, as transplant function deteriorates, there may be a requirement for other treatments used for patients with CKD.

Interesting facts

While the risk of many malignancies is increased in transplant recipients, no increased risk has been demonstrated with some cancers (including breast, prostate and rectum).

Interesting facts

Immunosuppressive therapy increases the risk of many infections. Post-transplant infections may also predispose to certain cancers (e.g. lymphomas associated with Epstein–Barr virus) and allograft dysfunction (e.g. BK virus).

Conservative therapy for advanced chronic kidney disease

In patients approaching ESKD for whom dialysis is unlikely to prolong survival or improve quality of life, such as older patients with significant comorbid conditions, 'conservative' treatment without dialysis should be considered. As optimal conservative therapy may be effective at prolonging quality of life, it should be directed not only at symptom control and avoiding acute deterioration, but also at delaying progression of CKD, reducing the complications of CKD and treating comorbid conditions (see Box 9.6).

Box 9.6 Principles of conservative therapy for advanced CKD without dialysis

Avoid nephrotoxins, unnecessary polypharmacy and contraindicated drugs
Optimize management of blood pressure and fluid status
Treat dangerous electrolyte abnormalities
Treat symptoms of uraemia
Consider continuation of therapy to slow CKD progression
Optimize social functioning, using a multidisciplinary approach
Plan for a calm and dignified death with minimal suffering

To prolong and improve quality of life, therapy should include avoidance of nephrotoxins (e.g. drugs, intravenous radiocontrast), regular assessment of all medications to avoid unnecessary polypharmacy and nephrotoxicity, avoidance or rapid reversal of AKI (e.g. from hypovolaemia or sepsis), treatment for specific symptoms of CKD, correction of dangerous electrolyte abnormalities, and specific measures to slow CKD progression.

Death from ESKD should be planned, peaceful and dignified. As long as severe symptoms (in particular fluid overload) are avoided, then suffering should be minimal and death occurs by progressive obtundation.

END-STAGE KIDNEY DISEASE AND REPLACEMENT OF RENAL FUNCTION

HYPERTENSION AND THE KIDNEY

10

Chapter objectives

After studying this chapter you should be able to:

1. List some physiological determinants of the arterial blood pressure and explain the role of the kidney in regulating these factors.

2. Discuss some mechanisms whereby abnormalities of the kidney may lead to hypertension (both essential and secondary forms).

3. Describe the pathology involved in end-organ damage due to hypertension.

4. Outline the principles of clinical and laboratory assessment of a patient presenting with hypertension.

5. Describe the mechanisms of action of the major classes of antihypertensive drugs.

6. Give the principles of management of a patient with renovascular hypertension.

Introduction

Arterial hypertension is the most prevalent chronic disorder of western populations. If untreated, it can result in a wide spectrum of morbidity and premature mortality and, as such, its prevention and treatment are major goals for health care systems.

The kidney is involved both as a causative factor and as an organ of target damage in hypertension, and this chapter will outline some of its physiological and pathological features in relation to hypertension. The subject is a very large one and the discussion here will necessarily be selective.

See Case 10.1:1.

Determinants of normal blood pressure and role of the kidney

In its simplest form, the haemodynamic description of the systemic circulation can be reduced to the statement that the mean arterial blood pressure (BP) is the product of the cardiac output (CO) and the total peripheral resistance (TPR), i.e.

$$BP = CO \times TPR$$

The cardiac output itself is the product of the stroke volume times the heart rate, where the stroke volume is determined by the left ventricular filling volume and the force of contraction. While a very wide range of physiological variables can influence blood pressure through one or other of these parameters, and the relationship between them is in fact very complex, these formulae suggest a number of levels at which the function of the kidney may impact upon the final level of the blood pressure. Some of these mechanisms are illustrated in Fig. 10.1.

The two main variables to be considered are the extracellular fluid volume (which relates directly to the cardiac output) and the degree of vasoconstriction of the arterial bed (which determines the total peripheral resistance). Many aspects of renal function impinge on one or both of these variables. The following are some examples.

- Anything causing a reduction of glomerular filtration rate (GFR) will lead to retention of salt and water, with consequent volume expansion.

- Excessive salt reabsorption by the renal tubules will also lead to increased extracellular fluid (ECF) volume.

- Activation of the renin–angiotensin–aldosterone system has the capacity to influence both variables: angiotensin II is a potent vasoconstrictor and also enhances proximal sodium reabsorption, while aldosterone stimulates distal nephron sodium reabsorption.

- The sympathetic nervous system likewise has dual actions: noradrenergic innervation of arteriolar vessels throughout the body leads to vasoconstriction and an increase in total peripheral resistance, while

---

Hypertension and the kidney: 1

A case of deteriorating blood pressure control

Ross Schneider is a 72-year-old man who presents to his local doctor with 3 weeks of increasing headaches. He also mentions having been generally unwell for several months, with tiredness and increasing breathlessness on exertion. He is known to have had mild hypertension for over 25 years, but his blood pressure has been well controlled over this period of time, his current medication being the diuretic indapamide 2.5 mg daily. However, he has been living overseas with his son for the past 9 months and, during this period, has not had his blood pressure checked as regularly as usual. His past history also includes peripheral vascular disease, manifested 2 years previously by episodes of **claudication** in both calves on walking up hills. This symptom had eased after he stopped smoking and no further investigation or treatment had been performed.

His family history includes hypertension in his father and one of his two sisters, and ischaemic heart disease which affected his father in his fifties. Mr Schneider is a retired postal officer who smoked about 20 cigarettes per day from age 20 to 70 years. He drinks four or five beers (300 mL glasses) per day. He takes no medications other than his blood pressure tablets and says he complies strictly with these.

On examination he looks rather tired and has a pulse rate of 90 beats/min. His blood pressure is 210/100, taken in the right arm in the seated position, and this is unchanged after 5 min of rest. The apex beat is found to be displaced 2 cm lateral to the mid-clavicular line, and is thrusting (pressure-loaded) in character. Cardiac auscultation reveals a systolic ejection murmur and a loud aortic component of the second heart sound. A few soft **crepitations** are heard in the base of both lung fields. The abdomen is normal to palpation but, on auscultating over the right upper quadrant, a prolonged systolic **bruit** is heard. Peripheral pulses are difficult to feel below the popliteal in both legs. The optic fundi show thickening of arteriolar walls and **arteriovenous nipping**. Urinalysis shows protein and no other abnormalities.

Two main issues arise for discussion from this presentation.

1. What was the basis of Mr Schneider's original history of hypertension?
2. What has occurred to cause his blood pressure control to be dramatically impaired at this presentation?

---

noradrenergic nerve endings around the proximal tubule stimulate sodium and water reabsorption at that site.

- The endothelium-derived peptide endothelin is a potent vasoconstrictor, and levels are elevated in renal failure.

- The renal prostaglandins are one of a number of locally acting signalling mechanisms influencing renal function in relation to hypertension. In this

Fig. 10.1 Renal mechanisms involved in blood pressure control. Note that many interactions exist between the factors included on this schematic diagram. While extracellular fluid (ECF) volume and vasoconstriction are shown here as independent parameters, there is direct interplay between these factors, as discussed in the text. GFR, glomerular filtration rate; NO, nitric oxide; PAF, platelet-activating factor; PG, prostaglandins; +indicates a stimulating or enhancing influence, −indicates an inhibiting or suppressing effect.

case, endproducts such as prostaglandin E_2 actually promote antihypertensive effects within the kidney, both by inhibiting salt and water reabsorption and hence promoting volume loss, and also by causing vasodilatation within the kidney and elsewhere.

- A number of other vasodilator systems have been identified within the kidney: these include a 'neutral lipid' identified in the renal medulla, the renal kinin system resulting in formation of the vasodilator bradykinin, as well as platelet-activating factor, nitric oxide and other endothelial-based dilator systems.

It is important to emphasize that there is no simple relationship between disturbances in these factors and the generation of sustained arterial hypertension. Perturbations in any one system tend to be compensated by changes in other systems, and the critical role of central nervous system pathways modulating baroreceptor reflexes must be taken into account. Furthermore, a primary change in one major parameter, such as the ECF, can lead to secondary changes in the state of peripheral vasoconstriction, so that the final pattern of haemodynamic disturbance is different from that which triggered the initial blood pressure rise.

Pathogenesis of essential hypertension

These considerations may be relevant to the pathogenesis of so-called 'essential' hypertension, in which a specific underlying cause for increased blood pressure cannot be defined in identifiable pathology in any organ system. This pattern, which would match the initial hypertensive history of our patient Mr Schneider, is associated with a family history of hypertension and the development of an increased blood pressure in the affected subject dur-

ing the third to fifth decade of life. While the precise pathogenesis of this condition has not been definitively established (and indeed a variety of physiological disturbances are capable of leading to the endpoint of sustained hypertension), one plausible scenario is shown in Fig. 10.2.

In this model, which is consistent with the findings of some clinical studies and a number of animal models, a primary inherited abnormality in renal salt retention is proposed, involving an overly avid sodium reabsorption mechanism in one or more segments of the nephron. This would lead to a phase of initial ECF volume expansion, which is later replaced by increased peripheral vasoconstriction and normalization of the ECF volume. One plausible mechanism whereby this haemodynamic change may occur involves the detection of the early volume expansion by volume receptors whose afferent signals into the central nervous system result in the release of a natriuretic hormone. Such a substance has been defined in the circulation during volume expansion, with properties like those of the natural **glycoside** ouabain, namely that it acts as an inhibitor of membrane-bound Na,K-ATPase. Inhibition of this enzyme in the renal tubules results in impaired sodium reabsorption and hence increased urinary excretion of salt and water, serving to correct the expanded ECF volume towards normal. However, inhibition of the same enzyme in smooth muscle cells within arteriolar walls results in an increase in intracellular sodium concentration which, by slowing the activity of a sodium–calcium exchanger in the muscle cell membrane, leads to an increase in intracellular calcium. This change triggers activation of the contractile mechanism of the smooth muscle fibres, leading to generalized vasoconstriction and an increase in total peripheral resistance, corresponding with the observed pattern of steady state haemodynamics in established hypertension.

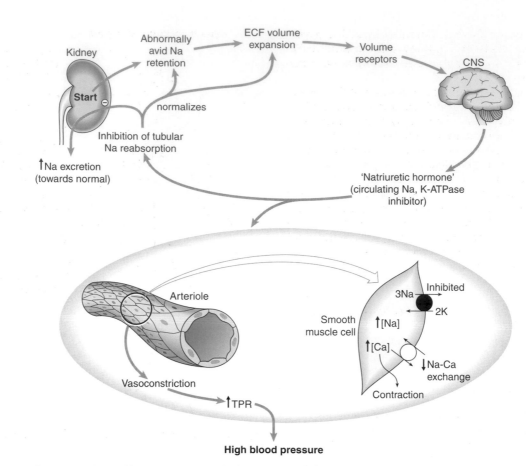

Fig. 10.2 Chronic volume expansion and hypertension: a model for essential hypertension? CNS, central nervous system; ECF, extracellular fluid; TPR, total peripheral resistance.

While speculative, the schema described above does accord with much of the available data about renal and circulatory changes observed during the generation and maintenance of hypertension. It also gives a framework for considering other factors known to predispose towards hypertension, whether or not there is another pathologically definable cause. A list of such risk factors is provided in Box 10.1.

Among the non-modifiable risk factors is a positive family history of hypertension. While this can not universally be associated at this stage with a specific genetic defect, a number of rare inherited syndromes have been defined which do fit in with the above model for essential hypertension involving primary renal volume retention. Of recent interest is the definition of the cause of hypertension in Liddle's syndrome, in which blood pressure elevation early in life is associated with evidence for volume expansion (suppressed renin and aldosterone levels). Here overexpression of the epithelial sodium channel in the apical membrane of the cortical collecting duct epithelium has been identified and linked to a specific gene defect. Similar but more subtle causes of increased tubular sodium avidity may underlie a wider spectrum of patients with familial hypertension. For

Box 10.1 Risk factors for development of high blood pressure (other than specific secondary forms of hypertension)

Non-modifiable

Family history
  Inherited predisposition to essential hypertension
  Specific inherited conditions (e.g. Liddle's syndrome, metabolic syndrome)

Potentially reversible

Lifestyle factors
  Obesity (± sleep apnoea)
  Excessive salt intake
  Excessive alcohol intake
  Physical inactivity
Iatrogenic
  Oral contraceptive pill use
  Use of non-steroidal anti-inflammatory drugs
  Steroid therapy
  Excessive use of topical or systemic vasoconstrictor medications

example, in the 'metabolic syndrome', in which hypertension is associated with obesity and insulin resistance, an increase in proximal tubular sodium–hydrogen exchange has been found.

Of the non-genetic factors, at least some of the reversible factors may operate through enhanced renal sodium retention. Certainly the epidemiological and clinical evidence relating to a correlation between salt intake and hypertension is suggestive of a primary role for volume expansion (at least in genetically predisposed individuals). The hypertension of common obesity may also be caused by volume expansion, possibly mediated by high insulin levels which act to enhance proximal sodium reabsorption. Renal salt retention is also implicated in the hypertension associated with a variety of medications, including oestrogens, non-steroidal anti-inflammatory drugs which interfere with prostaglandin synthesis, and corticosteroids.

ECF volume expansion also has an important role in the genesis of a number of forms of secondary hypertension; these are discussed later in this chapter.

Interesting facts

The epidemic of hypertension in modern human populations may relate to our evolutionary past as a species. Since our early terrestrial evolution occurred largely in salt-poor regions of the world such as Africa, physiological systems developed which were salt-avid. Hence when dietary salt is plentiful in the modern world, particularly in the West, salt retention occurs leading to volume expansion and hypertension.

The pathology of hypertension

Whatever the cause of a sustained increase in arterial blood pressure, a number of forms of end-organ damage result from this haemodynamic change. As shown in Fig. 10.3, the kidneys are included among these target organs.

The fundamental pathology associated with hypertension is based on structural changes in the terminal radicals of the arterial tree, namely the small muscular arteries and arterioles. The repetitive mechanical stress associated with hypertension causes changes in all layers of the vessel wall, particularly in the media layer, where smooth muscle hypertrophy results in a thickening of the arterial wall with concentric narrowing of the lumen. The internal elastic lamina becomes reduplicated and interrupted, and hyaline degeneration may occur in focal areas of the media where a glassy eosinophilic material accumulates. These changes, found in so-called 'benign' hypertension, are replaced in the more accelerated and severe variant known as 'malignant'

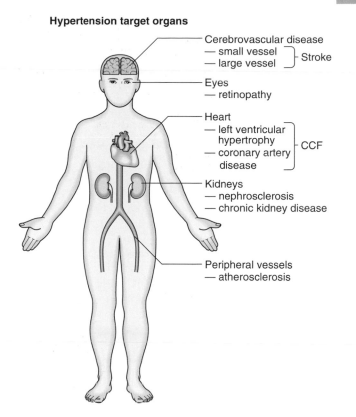

Hypertension target organs

Cerebrovascular disease
— small vessel
— large vessel } Stroke

Eyes
— retinopathy

Heart
— left ventricular hypertrophy
— coronary artery disease } CCF

Kidneys
— nephrosclerosis
— chronic kidney disease

Peripheral vessels
— atherosclerosis

Fig. 10.3 End-organ damage in hypertension. CCF, congestive cardiac failure.

hyper-tension by a more destructive severe form of vascular wall pathology, the characteristic lesion being that of fibrinoid necrosis. In all forms of sustained hypertension, the intima layer is also damaged and undergoes a proliferative response, which in larger vessels is associated with acceleration of the process of **atherosclerosis**.

These vascular lesions lead to various grades of ischaemia in the principal target organs, namely the brain, the heart and the kidneys. Small vessel changes in the brain are reflected in the optic fundi, where progressive stages of vascular damage and retinal ischaemia can be observed directly (hypertensive retinopathy). In the heart, myocardial ischaemia develops, and is aggravated by the development of left ventricular hypertrophy as a result of the chronic pressure load on that chamber. Within the kidney, ischaemia is manifested initially by wrinkling of the glomerular basement membrane. Hypertrophic and hyaline changes develop in the afferent arterioles, resulting in progressive atrophy and ultimately sclerosis of glomeruli (Fig. 10.4). In severe and neglected hypertension this can lead to end-stage kidney disease, a not uncommon outcome despite current antihypertensive treatment (see Chapter 8). Ischaemic changes also affect the tubules, which undergo atrophy,

Fig. 10.4 Microscopic pathology of the kidney in 'benign' essential hypertension. Note (a) the hypertrophied arterial walls and (b) hyaline degeneration of the afferent arteriole . One glomerulus (c) has undergone ischaemic contraction and there is interstitial fibrosis and inflammation (d).

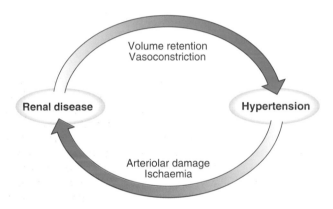

Fig. 10.5 The kidney in hypertension: both villain (cause) and victim (effect).

associated with interstitial inflammatory changes progressing ultimately to fibrosis. Eventually the kidney as a whole undergoes contraction with a finely scarred surface ('nephrosclerosis').

It is clear that the kidney has an especially complex relationship to arterial hypertension. As mentioned previously (and to be developed further below), it is directly implicated in the aetiology and pathophysiology of some forms of hypertension, notably those in which definable renal disease provides the primary trigger for the development of high blood pressure. Equally, however, it is an important end-organ of damage from hypertensive vascular disease, thereby setting up a vicious cycle of further aggravation of the hypertension (Fig. 10.5). Intervention in this cycle by vigorous therapy to lower the blood pressure and protect the kidney is thus a crucial task for clinicians caring for these patients.

See 10.1: 2.

Case 10.1 Hypertension and the kidney: 2

Initial investigations

Mr Schneider's physical examination (see 10.1: 1) revealed clear evidence for end-organ damage consistent with hypertensive effects. The displaced and prominent left ventricular impulse suggests the presence of left ventricular hypertrophy with some cardiac enlargement, and the pulmonary crepitations and recent history of breathlessness are consistent with early left ventricular failure. The history of claudication and finding of poor distal pulses in the legs suggest the development of peripheral vascular disease, while the finding of Grade II hypertensive retinopathy (thickened retinal arteriolar walls and arteriovenous nipping) implies hypertensive effects on small arterioles. The detection of proteinuria on urinalysis is consistent with hypertensive damage to glomeruli.

The initial investigations performed on Mr Schneider reveal the following results:

Plasma biochemistry:
Sodium 135 mmol/L
Potassium 4.1 mmol/L
Chloride 99 mmol/L
Bicarbonate 29 mmol/L
*Urea 9.2 mmol/L
*Creatinine 0.18 mmol/L.

These levels had been normal when last checked 3 years previously.

Random blood glucose is 6.8 mmol/L and the lipid profile is normal. A chest X-ray shows a moderately enlarged heart (principally the left ventricle) and bilateral pulmonary congestion. Electrocardiography shows evidence of left ventricular hypertrophy with non-specific ST segment changes.

These data were interpreted as evidence for renal and cardiac damage resulting from his hypertension.

While waiting for these initial investigation results, Mr Schneider's doctor initiated some changes in his therapy, having made the assessment that he had experienced a marked deterioration in his level of blood pressure control. He urged the patient to discontinue all alcohol intake, to reduce his salt intake, to continue with his diuretic medication and to commence taking prazosin 2 mg three times daily. He asked to review him in 3 days time. He explained that he suspected that some new problem had arisen causing his hypertension to become exacerbated, and that he thought some further investigations would be required.

Issues for further consideration at this point include:

1. What clues are there as to the cause of Mr Schneider's deterioration in blood pressure control?
2. What are the appropriate next steps in his management?

*Values outside the normal range; see Appendix.

Table 10.1 Overview of main classes of antihypertensive drugs

Class	Prototype drug(s)	Advantages	Disadvantages
Diuretics	Chlorothiazide	Useful in coexistent CCF, adjunctive action with other agents	Electrolyte/metabolic side effects, allergies
Beta-blockers	Metoprolol (beta-1 selective)	Beneficial in IHD	Fatigue, insomnia; may worsen asthma, heart block, PVD, lipids
Alpha-blockers	Prazosin	Metabolically neutral	Postural hypotension
Calcium channel blockers*	(a) Verapamil (b) Nifedipine	All useful in angina (best used in slow-release preparations)	(a) May cause constipation, worsen heart block/CCF; (b) Cause flushing, oedema
ACE inhibitors	Captopril	Beneficial in CCF, reduce proteinuria, conserve K	Cough, angio-oedema, reduce GFR in renal artery stenosis
A-II receptor blockers	Losartan	As for ACE inhibitors, but less cough	
Centrally acting drugs	Methyldopa, clonidine		Drowsiness, depression
Direct acting vasodilators	Hydralazine, minoxidil		Reflex tachycardia, oedema

ACE, angiotensin-converting enzyme; A II, angiotensin II; CCF, congestive cardiac failure; GFR, glomerular filtration rate; IHD, ischaemic heart disease; PVD, peripheral vascular disease.

*Representative drugs are shown for the two main classes of calcium channel blockers: (a) the non-dihydropyridines; and (b) the dihydropyridines.

Principles in the management of hypertension

In a patient presenting for the first time with hypertension, management consists of three general steps:

1. Confirmation of the persistence of hypertension on multiple observations following modification of reversible lifestyle factors (see Box 10.1).

2. Baseline investigations to assess end-organ damage (particularly in the heart and kidney), to quantitate other vascular risk factors (particularly plasma lipid profile), and to screen for major causes of secondary hypertension as clinically appropriate (see below).

3. Initiation of pharmacological treatment.

This staged approach can be accelerated in situations in which the blood pressure is severely elevated at presentation (>160/100) or where there is clinical evidence of organ-threatening complications such as heart failure, renal impairment or neurological symptoms or signs. In practice, in the absence of specific clinical clues, the 'screening' investigations in the second step can be limited to urinalysis to detect renal parenchymal disease and plasma biochemistry to detect renal failure or electrolyte changes suggestive of endocrine hypertension. Further investigations are initiated when abnormalities are detected on these preliminary tests, taken in conjunction with clinical information.

The selection of an appropriate antihypertensive medication depends on properties of the available agents (including cost), patient characteristics and co-morbid conditions, guided by information from relevant published clinical trials. A brief summary of some key features of the available drugs is given in Table 10.1. The most commonly used agents are currently from two classes, the calcium-channel blockers, and drugs interfering with the renin–angiotensin system, including ACE inhibitors and A-II receptor blockers (the recently developed renin inhibitors also belong to this group). Frequently, drugs are given in combination to reduce side effects and oppose secondary compensations which can reduce the effectiveness of a single agent. One of the most effective such combinations is a low dose diuretic together with an ACE inhibitor or A-II receptor blocker.

Interesting facts

Before the middle of the 20th century, hypertension was commonly ascribed to an over-excited emotional state, and treatments usually included central nervous system sedatives such as barbiturates.

Deterioration in blood pressure control

When a patient who has been stabilized on an antihypertensive treatment regimen experiences a deterioration in blood pressure control, as did Mr Schneider, a number of possibilities must be considered (Box 10.2). The patient's adherence to the recommended treatment regimen must always be checked since poor compliance is a relatively frequent phenomenon, especially when the medications used are associated with unwelcome side effects. Occasionally, the inadvertent coprescription of an interacting

Box 10.2 Causes of deterioration in blood pressure control

Poor treatment adherence (compliance)
Commencement of interacting medications (e.g. NSAIDs)
Lifestyle changes (weight gain, excessive salt or alcohol intake)
Superadded secondary hypertension (especially renovascular or renal parenchymal disease)

NSAIDs, non-steroidal anti-inflammatory drugs.

Fig. 10.6 Principal causes of secondary hypertension.

medication may be the cause; the best example here is commencement of a non-steroidal anti-inflammatory drug which promotes salt and water retention and will elevate the blood pressure in predisposed individuals. Occasionally, there has been a progressive slide into poor lifestyle habits which raise the blood pressure, such as weight gain beyond ideal body weight or excess intake of salt or alcohol.

An important consideration in an older patient, however, is the possibility that a form of secondary hypertension has become superimposed on what was originally essential hypertension.

Secondary hypertension

The principal causes of secondary hypertension are illustrated in Fig. 10.6. One of these causes may be defined soon after presentation in a patient with newly diagnosed hypertension, or following a period of resistance to therapy or deterioration in blood pressure control in a patient with established hypertension. It should be emphasized that less than 10% of all hypertensive patients have hypertension secondary to a defined pathology in a specific organ system, although a higher percentage of underlying causes can be reported from clinics seeing a patient group referred for further investigation of 'difficult hypertension'. While causes other than those shown in Fig. 10.6 need to be considered in special patient groups (e.g. coarctation of the aorta in hypertensive children and pre-eclampsia in pregnant women), the most commonly encountered causes of secondary hypertension arise from conditions in the adrenal gland or the kidney.

Adrenal causes

Adrenal lesions causing hypertension may arise either in the adrenal cortex or medulla.

The adrenal cortex can be the site of an aldosterone-secreting adenoma, resulting in primary aldosteronism, or Conn's syndrome. In this condition autonomous production of aldosterone by the tumour leads to sustained salt and water retention by the kidney, with volume expansion and secondary vasoconstriction which sustains

the hypertensive state, as previously discussed. Frequently, this condition is accompanied by hypokalaemia, reflecting the action of aldosterone in enhancing renal potassium excretion. While a low serum potassium, usually accompanied by an elevated bicarbonate concentration, may act as a useful clue to the presence of an aldosterone excess state, these electrolyte abnormalities are not universally found in cases of primary aldosterone overproduction, and some authorities recommend screening for this condition in all patients whose hypertension is resistant to usual treatment. One screening approach depends on the measurement of plasma aldosterone and renin concentrations, using a high aldosterone:renin ratio as a signal for further adrenal investigation. Primary aldosteronism can also arise from hyperplasia of both adrenal cortices, sometimes because of an inherited defect in adrenal corticosteroid biosynthesis.

When the adrenal adenoma or cortical hypertrophy is associated with autonomous secretion of the glucocorticoid hormone cortisol, Cushing's syndrome results, hypertension being one of the principal clinical manifestations. Other clues here are bodily **habitus** changes associated with glucocorticoid excess, accompanied by hyperglycaemia as well as hypokalaemia and alkalosis (see also *Systems of the Body: The Endocrine System*).

The adrenal medulla may also give rise to tumours causing hypertension, in this case phaeochromocytoma, secreting the catecholamines adrenaline (epinephrine), noradrenaline (norepinephrine) and related metabolites. These tumours can also arise in neural crest-derived tissue outside the adrenal gland. Characteristically they are associated with labile hypertension, with spasms of vasoconstriction and organ ischaemia related to bursts of catecholamine release. However, a significant proportion of these tumours are accompanied by sustained hypertension without such dramatic episodic changes in the peripheral circulation. Investigation is based on an index

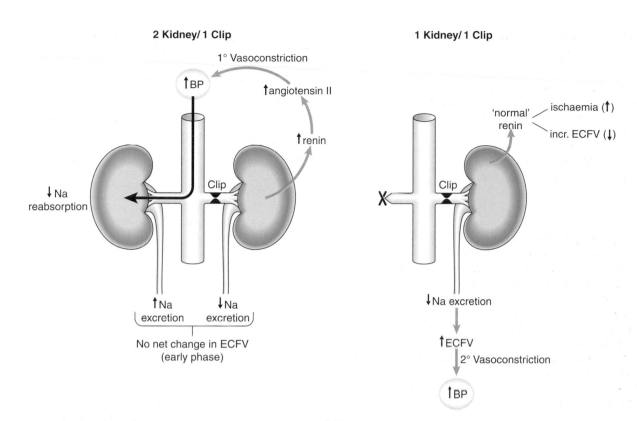

2 Kidney/ 1 Clip

1° Vasoconstriction

↑BP

↑angiotensin II

↑renin

Clip

↓Na reabsorption

↑Na excretion   ↓Na excretion

No net change in ECFV (early phase)

1 Kidney/ 1 Clip

'normal' renin

ischaemia (↑)

incr. ECFV (↓)

X   Clip

↓Na excretion

↑ECFV

2° Vasoconstriction

↑BP

Fig. 10.7 Pathophysiology of renovascular hypertension (Goldblatt models). The two experimental models shown here represent extreme illustrations of the role of vasoconstriction (early phase of two kidney/one clip model) and volume expansion (one kidney/one clip) in the generation of hypertension during renal ischaemia (see text for details). BP, blood pressure; ECFV, extracellular fluid volume.

of suspicion, leading to 24 h urine collections for measurement of catecholamines and their metabolites, followed by CT imaging of the adrenal gland. Radioisotope scans with specialized tracers (e.g. MIBG; *meta*-iodobenzguanine) can be useful in localizing extra-adrenal phaeochromocytomas. The pathophysiology of the hypertension in this condition relates to intense catecholamine-induced vasoconstriction rather than primary volume expansion. The cornerstone of treatment before operative removal of the tumour is effective alpha-blockade using agents such as phenoxybenzamine.

Renal causes

The kidney can be the cause of secondary hypertension by one of two fundamental mechanisms: via activation of the renin–angiotensin system in renal ischaemia due to renovascular disease, or through non-renin-dependent mechanisms in renal parenchymal disease, both in its early stages and in end-stage renal failure.

The mechanisms involved in the various forms of renal hypertension are best illuminated through some classic experiments first performed by Goldblatt over 60 years ago (Fig. 10.7).

When the renal artery supplying one kidney of an animal is clipped so that the lumen is reduced by more than 70%, the animal develops hypertension. The mechanism of the initial phase of blood pressure rise is dependent on the activation of secretion of renin from the clipped kidney, largely because of the fall in perfusion pressure in the afferent arterioles beyond the obstructed artery (see Chapter 2). Within the first few weeks after production of this lesion, the blood pressure can be normalized by agents interfering with the action of angiotensin II, verifying that vasoconstriction produced by this peptide is the main mechanism for the hypertension. The ECF volume does not undergo significant change in this phase, partly because the reduction in sodium excretion from the clipped kidney is compensated by an increase in sodium excretion from the unclipped kidney. This is because of the effect of the increased blood pressure in the unclipped kidney to inhibit salt and water reabsorption in proximal tubules on that side (so-called 'pressure natriuresis'). After some months, however, the increased blood pressure becomes resistant to the action of angiotensin inhibition, but does respond to a reduction of ECF volume. This is because of the long-term effects of sustained hypertension on the blood vessels of the unclipped kidney, where obliterative changes lead to glomerular damage and reduced excretion of salt and water from that side. That is, the initial vasoconstriction-mediated hypertension has been replaced by a volume-dependent pattern.

When a similar experiment is performed in an animal in which one of the kidneys has been removed, clipping the renal artery of the remaining kidney also leads to development of hypertension, but in this case both the early phase and the longer term phase of hypertension are dependent on an expanded ECF volume. This is because, despite the ischaemia which would otherwise trigger renin release, the overall reduction in total GFR means that volume retention occurs early in the model, counteracting the stimulus for renin release and triggering hypertension through secondary vasoconstriction via mechanisms described earlier in this chapter. This model provides a basis for understanding the hypertension of advanced renal insufficiency ('renoprival' hypertension), in which volume expansion is nearly always present.

Renal artery stenosis

Renal artery stenosis occurs in man in one of two main pathological forms.

Fibromuscular dysplasia is a congenital condition in which the development of the media or adventitia layer of the renal artery (and sometimes other arteries) is abnormal, leading to an irregular narrowing of the lumen, often in a 'beaded' pattern. Typically affecting young women in the second or third decade of life, this is one of the classic causes of secondary hypertension in a young patient and, when unilateral, is usually detected in the phase of high renin release from the affected kidney, corresponding to the initial phase of two kidney/ one clip Goldblatt hypertension. Surgical intervention to correct the stenosis frequently results in restoration of normal blood pressure and protection of renal function.

The more common cause of renal artery stenosis is that due to atherosclerosis, affecting patients in older age groups. In this condition the atherosclerotic pathology, which may also affect other vascular beds, involves one or both renal arteries, frequently producing a relatively focal stenosis (Fig. 10.8). While there is often no special clue to the presence of this underlying lesion, the clinician's index of suspicion that stenosis is present is raised by the following:

- The relatively sudden appearance of hypertension in an older person.

- The development of resistance to usual antihypertensive medications or an abrupt deterioration in blood pressure control in a patient with previously stable hypertension (as in our current case).

- Severe hypertension in an older patient associated with progressive deterioration of renal function.

Careful clinical, biochemical and radiological analysis is necessary to define the presence of renal artery stenosis in selected patients, and the pathophysiological assessment and appropriate management of such patients is frequently a complex matter. Three basic components are involved in the overall assessment:

- What is the morphology of the lesions in the renal artery (or arteries)?

- What is the role of the renal artery stenosis in the pathogenesis of the patient's hypertension at this time?

- What is the influence of the renal arterial disease on overall renal function?

A number of imaging modalities, summarized in Table 10.2, may be used to define the anatomy of the renal arteries. While intra-arterial digital subtraction arteriography (Fig. 10.8) is the gold standard for definition of renal artery lesions, recent technical advances have made alternative less invasive procedures such as magnetic resonance angiography attractive alternatives.

Fig. 10.8 Intra-arterial digital subtraction arteriogram showing atheromatous renal artery stenosis on the left side in a 60-year-old woman with severe hypertension.

Table 10.2 Methods of renal artery imaging

Technique	Comments
Digital subtraction angiography	Intra-arterial method provides gold standard; intravenous approach lacks adequate resolution
	Requires use of contrast agent (may reduce GFR)
Spiral CT angiography	Good 3D images; uses intravenous contrast (often high volumes required)
Magnetic resonance angiography	Avoids contrast agent; accurate only for main (proximal) vessels, expensive, limited availability
Renal artery Doppler–ultrasound scan	Operator-dependent; variable sensitivity/specificity
Radionuclide renography with captopril	Poor anatomical resolution but sensitive detection of functional stenosis via GFR effects

GFR, glomerular filtration rate.

One procedure which gives poor anatomical definition but potentially useful functional information is the captopril renogram. The uptake of a tracer isotope by both kidneys is compared before and after administration of a single dose of the angiotensin-converting enzyme (ACE) inhibitor captopril. The rationale for this test depends on the fact that, in the ischaemic kidney, the GFR in individual nephrons is maintained by the vasoconstrictor action of locally produced angiotensin II on the efferent arteriole. Thus, reduction of angiotensin II synthesis by captopril leads to an abrupt fall in tracer filtration in the kidney affected by significant renal artery stenosis. The sensitivity of this test is reduced in the presence of renal impairment.

The functional effect of the stenosis can be indirectly assessed by comparing the renin concentration in blood samples taken directly from the renal vein draining each kidney: an increase in renal vein renin on the affected side of greater than 1.5 times the contralateral kidney is suggestive of significant ischaemia. While this investigation has some capacity to predict the renin dependence of hypertension in the early phase of renovascular hypertension, its utility is limited, both by technical factors and because hypertensive vascular disease has frequently supervened in the unstenosed kidney by the time many such patients are investigated (equivalent to the late phase of two kidney/one clip Goldblatt hypertension). Indeed, intervention to improve the blood flow into kidneys affected by atherosclerotic renal artery stenosis is sometimes justified by the need to preserve long-term renal function, regardless of the mechanism by which the renal artery disease has contributed to the patient's hypertension.

Renal parenchymal disease

Hypertension in renal parenchymal disease has multiple possible origins. In the phase before advanced loss of renal function has occurred, one important factor may be the loss of vasodilator substances generated normally by healthy renal tissue (including the 'neutral lipid' from the renal medulla). This may lead to unopposed systemic vasoconstriction. However, as renal functional impairment progresses, the dominant mechanism is undoubtedly retention of salt and water as a result of the inadequate GFR, leading to expansion of the ECF volume and hypertension through secondary vasoconstrictive mechanisms (discussed previously). Thus, the great majority of patients approaching end-stage kidney disease, or on dialysis, have volume-dependent hypertension which can be difficult to control until salt and water are removed from the ECF by diuretics or a form of dialysis.

In a minority of patients with advanced renal disease (<10%), the pathological processes within the kidney cause it to act as an ongoing source of renin release, producing hypertension via angiotensin-induced vasoconstriction. In individual patients, activation of the sympathetic nervous system appears to play a role in the pathogenesis of hypertension in renal failure, and in

---

Case 10.1 — Hypertension and the kidney: 3

Further investigations and management

Three factors in Mr Schneider's case led his doctor to initiate further investigation for renal artery stenosis. First, a bruit over the upper abdomen had been heard on clinical examination, suggestive (but not diagnostic) of critical narrowing in a renal artery or other branch of the abdominal aorta. Second, he had recently developed clinical evidence for significant peripheral vascular disease, suggestive of a widespread process of advanced atherosclerosis. Third, his serum creatinine had risen over recent years, suggesting some cause of impaired glomerular perfusion.

After referral to a consultant nephrologist, a number of further studies were performed which confirmed this suspicion. A renal ultrasound demonstrated that the right kidney was 3cm smaller in longitudinal axis than the left kidney, and a renal artery Doppler ultrasound study indicated wave forms consistent with stenosis near the origin of the right renal artery. A radionuclide scan indicated reduced uptake and excretion of tracer on the right side, with a further drop in right-sided perfusion after a 25mg dose of captopril.

With these preliminary data in hand, Mr Schneider went on to undergo an intra-arterial digital subtraction angiogram of his renal arteries. A 90% stenosis in the proximal segment of the right renal artery was demonstrated, with only minor luminal irregularities in the left renal artery, but significant atheromatous disease in the abdominal aorta. At the same procedure, the right renal artery lesion was dilated by balloon angioplasty and a short metallic **stent** was implanted to maintain luminal patency at the end of the procedure. Mr Schneider tolerated the procedure well. The day after this intervention his plasma creatinine rose to *0.23mmol/L, but over the next few weeks it fell to a value of *0.15mmol/L, where it remained for several months of follow-up. His blood pressure became rather easier to control, although it still required the coadministration of indapamide plus prazosin 1mg b.d.

*Values outside the normal range; see Appendix.

---

these cases high circulating levels of catecholamines are found. See 10.1: 3.

While the precise pathophysiology involved in the hypertension associated with renovascular disease is rarely defined clearly in an individual patient, the pattern illustrated by Mr Schneider's case is fairly characteristic of the situation in atherosclerotic renal artery stenosis. While ischaemia and renin release may be involved relatively early in the pathological process, the contralateral kidney is soon affected by hypertensive arteriolar disease, superimposed on any pre-existing vascular or parenchymal changes (this is a major cause of the fall in GFR in this clinical setting). Thus, while correction of the renal artery stenosis cannot be expected to cure the hypertension altogether, it can result in improved ability to control the blood pressure (reduced medication requirements), and may help to preserve renal function both in the kidney affected by the stenosis and also in the contralateral kidney through better blood pressure control. While the risks associated with open surgical procedures to improve renal artery flow (bypass grafting or endarterectomy) can make the decision to intervene difficult, more recent closed procedures involving balloon angioplasty with stent placement have made intervention more viable for a larger number of patients.

PREGNANCY AND THE KIDNEY

Chapter objectives

After studying this chapter you should be able to:

1. Describe the anatomical changes that occur in the renal tract in normal pregnancy.

2. Understand the importance of diagnosis and treatment of urinary infection in pregnancy.

3. Demonstrate an understanding of the physiological alterations in pregnancy in fluid volume, renal plasma flow, glomerular filtration rate and blood pressure, and the mechanisms by which they occur.

4. Describe the 'normal' changes in plasma biochemistry seen during pregnancy and the mechanisms that underpin these changes.

5. Define the various categories of hypertensive disorders encountered in pregnant women.

6. Describe the systemic abnormalities that occur in pre-eclampsia.

7. Demonstrate an understanding of the approach to the management of hypertension in pregnancy.

Introduction

The renal system undergoes several important structural and functional changes during normal pregnancy. These have implications for understanding a number of common complications of pregnancy, as well as interpreting the results of laboratory and imaging investigations during pregnancy.

This chapter will survey these changes and introduce some important complications of pregnancy relating to the urinary tract, including the hypertensive disorders of pregnancy.

Structural changes in the urinary tract during pregnancy

Pregnancy induces changes in almost every organ system of the body, generally as an adaptive process to provide the best outcome for both mother and fetus. A key factor in supporting placental blood flow is the expansion of maternal blood volume which leads to increased cardiac output. As a consequence of the increased intra- and extravascular volume, the kidneys enlarge by up to 70%. However the most striking anatomical change in the urinary tract during pregnancy is dilatation of the pelvicalyceal system and the ureters (see Fig. 11.1). Generally the right side is affected more than the left. These changes develop in the first trimester and progress such that by the third trimester more than 90% of women will have dilated ureters and pelvicalyceal systems. The changes persist for up to 3 months post-partum. Hence images of the kidneys in the first 3 months post-partum should be interpreted with caution.

In general, these anatomical changes are completely asymptomatic. However, a small number of women will develop transient loin pain which may sometimes be severe. However the urine is sterile and few or no red blood cells are observed. Treatment should be expectant as symptoms will generally resolve post-partum.

The cause of the dilated urinary tract is debated. Some obstruction of the urinary drainage system occurs at the pelvic brim where the enlarged uterus may cause partial ureteric compression. Engorged vessels, for example a dilated ovarian venous plexus, uterine veins or iliac vessels, may also contribute to ureteric obstruction. Hormonal changes, including increases in oestrogen, progesterone, prostaglandins and relaxin, may also decrease smooth muscle contractility in the urinary tract and promote dilatation. The dilatation of the urinary tract in pregnancy contributes to the increased incidence of asymptomatic bacteriuria and pyelonephritis in pregnant women due to impaired urine drainage and the resultant urinary stasis.

The dilated urinary tract also contributes to a considerable 'dead space' if timed urine volumes are measured. Hence 24-hour urine collections are now rarely undertaken in pregnant patients because a sizeable and unquantifiable error will exist.

Case 11.1 Urinary tract infection in pregnancy: 1

Anne Farrell is a 26-year-old woman who presents in her first pregnancy at 8 weeks gestation for her first antenatal review. She has previously been well, apart from a history of recurrent urinary infection in her late teenage years. These had occurred at the time she began to be sexually active. They were generally treated with short courses of antibiotics. She had no episodes of upper urinary tract infection. No radiological investigations of her urinary tract had been performed. However, her renal function was determined to be normal.

Her only recent symptom has been some urinary frequency which she ascribed to early pregnancy, but she has not experienced dysuria. On examination in the clinic, her blood pressure is 95/60 mm Hg, pulse rate 96/minute, and urinalysis demonstrates blood, nitrites and leucocytes. Examination is otherwise normal. A midstream urine (MSU) examination is reported to show $10–100 \times 10^6$/L erythrocytes and $>100 \times 10^6$/L leucocytes, with a bacterial count of $>10^8$/L and a pure growth of *Escherichia coli* sensitive to both ampicillin and cephalosporins.

Having found an asymptomatic urinary infection in this pregnant patient, we should consider the normal anatomical changes that occur in the renal system during pregnancy that may predispose to complications such as urinary tract infection.

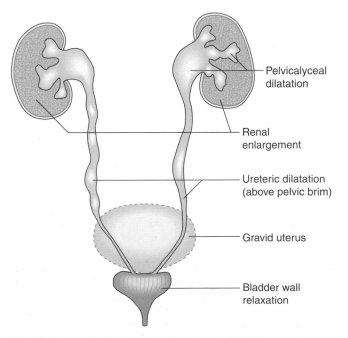

Fig. 11.1 Anatomical changes in the urinary tract during pregnancy.

- Pelvicalyceal dilatation
- Renal enlargement
- Ureteric dilatation (above pelvic brim)
- Gravid uterus
- Bladder wall relaxation

Case 11.1 Urinary tract infection in pregnancy: 2

Initial treatment

Anne is treated for one week with cephalexin 500 mg qid. One week later her MSU reveals a further *E. coli* infection, still sensitive to cephalosporins. She remains asymptomatic and is concerned about the possible effects of both infection and antibiotics on the pregnancy and her unborn child.

This raises the questions:

- What are the risks of untreated asymptomatic bacteriuria in pregnancy?
- How should recurrent infection in pregnancy be treated?
- What are the preferred antibiotics to use in pregnancy?

Urinary tract infection in pregnancy

Urinary infection has been associated with pre-eclampsia, pre-term delivery, increased caesarean section rates and intrauterine growth retardation. Hence detection and treatment of urinary infection in pregnancy is mandatory.

Collection of a clean sample of mid-stream urine is particularly problematic in pregnancy. Furthermore, an increased excretion of leucocytes occurs physiologically in pregnancy. Hence pyuria can be present without necessarily signifying infection.

Between 2% and 10% of women have *asymptomatic bacteriuria*, the incidence being similar in the pregnant and non-pregnant population. During pregnancy, 40% of untreated patients with asymptomatic bacteriuria will develop an acute symptomatic infection. Hence treatment is recommended. The choice of drug is determined by the sensitivity of the organism. Cephalosporins or ampicillin/amoxycillin are generally used as first-line agents. A single course of antibiotics is recommended with a follow-up urine culture one week later, and then at 4 weekly intervals throughout the pregnancy. Up to 25% of patients will relapse during the pregnancy and of these less than 5% will have their infection cleared by a further course of therapy. If not cleared by a second course of antibiotics, in general patients should be treated with a prophylactic nightly dose of antibiotic, either ampicillin or a cephalosporin, for the duration of the pregnancy.

Acute cystitis occurs in approximately 2% of pregnancies, the majority of infections occurring in women who are negative on an initial urine screen. Symptoms are similar to those occurring in non-pregnant women, but as pregnancy itself can also be associated with frequency, the symptoms can be misinterpreted. Treatment and follow-up are the same as for asymptomatic bacteriuria.

Acute pyelonephritis is more likely to follow from lower urinary tract infection in pregnant compared to non-pregnant women, due to the anatomical changes observed in the urinary tract in pregnancy. Symptoms are identical to those observed in non-pregnant patients. Treatment is dictated by the severity of the illness, and may include rehydration and parenteral antibiotics. In general, ampicillin/amoxycillin and cephalosporins are also used to treat pyelonephritis, but if bacteraemia occurs then aminoglycosides are recommended, with careful monitoring of blood levels. Renal imaging is often difficult to interpret due to the normal anatomical changes in pregnancy, and thus should generally be deferred until at least 3 months post-partum in patients with recurrent infection or pyelonephritis.

In choosing an antibiotic for use during pregnancy, sulfonamides should be avoided, particularly in the last four weeks of pregnancy, due to the increased risk of newborn hyperbilirubinaemia and kernicterus. Nitrofurantoin should also be avoided in the latter stages of pregnancy as it may be associated with neonatal haemolysis. Trimethoprim–sulfonamide combinations and tetracyclines should not be used throughout the pregnancy because of possible teratogenicity and the effects on teeth and bones respectively. There have been few studies using quinolones in pregnancy, but as these drugs have been documented to cause arthropathy in immature animals of various species, they should be avoided in pregnancy.

Case 11.1 Urinary tract infection in pregnancy: 3

Further treatment and outcome

Anne was treated for 10 days on this occasion with ampicillin 500 mg qid. However, one week later her MSU again demonstrated a pure growth of *E. coli*. Hence, following a further 10 days course of treatment, this time with cephalexin 500 mg qid, she was asked to take 500 mg cephalexin nocte as a prophylactic measure for the remainder of her pregnancy. Monthly MSUs did not show any recurrence and she delivered at term without complication. At review 3 months post-partum, she had no evidence of urinary tract infection and a renal ultrasound was normal.

Renal physiology changes in pregnancy

Changes in fluid volume during pregnancy

Approximately 10–14 kg of weight gain occurs in normal pregnancy, which is primarily due to an increase of 7–9 litres of water of which 6–7 litres is estimated to be extravascular and 2 litres intravascular. Plasma volume expansion starts in the first trimester, peaks at 32 weeks and continues till term. Hence hypervolaemia is present

Box 11.1 Factors influencing Na excretion during pregnancy

Decreased Na excretion	Increased Na excretion
Increased tubular Na reabsorption (via glomerulotubular balance)	Increase in GFR
	Hormones promoting Na loss:
Increased Na-retaining hormones:	Progesterone
Aldosterone	Vasopressin
Deoxycorticosteroid	Oxytocin
Oestrogens	Prostaglandins
Prolactin	Natriuretic hormone
Renin/angiotensin	Melanocyte stimulating hormone
Human placental lactogen	
Physical factors:	Physical factors:
Increase in ureteric pressure	Decreased serum albumin
Ureteroplacental shunt	Decrease in renal vascular resistance
Exaggerated influence of posture	

The net effect of these changes is considerable net retention of Na.

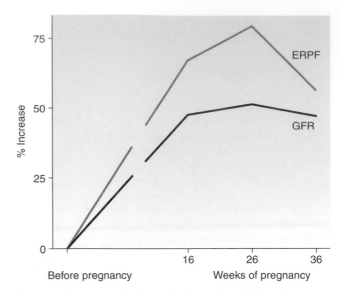

Fig 11.2 Changes in effective renal plasma flow (ERPF) and glomerular filtration rate (GFR) during pregnancy.

and results in an enhanced cardiac output of about 30–40% above pre-pregnant levels, which supports placental perfusion. Interstitial fluid volume also increases due to decreased oncotic pressure, consequent on a low serum albumin concentration secondary to dilution. Approximately 950 mmol of Na are retained in normal pregnancy, due to the net effect of the many haemodynamic, hormonal and physical changes that occur. These are summarized in Box 11.1.

Changes in renal plasma flow and glomerular filtration rate

In the normal pregnant woman, the effective renal plasma flow increases by up to 80% from conception to mid-pregnancy, and then falls in the third trimester to 50–60% above baseline (see Fig. 11.2). Glomerular filtration rate is increased by about 50% at the end of the first trimester and is maintained at that level till about 36 weeks gestation when it again falls to pre-pregnancy levels. As a result of the increased GFR, plasma urea and creatinine fall. Thus a plasma creatinine regarded as 'normal' in a non-pregnant individual may signify renal impairment in a pregnant person. The calculation of GFR by the MDRD formula (see Chapter 5) has been reported to significantly underestimate GFR in pregnancy and hence should not be used to monitor renal function.

Osmoregulation in pregnancy

Very early in pregnancy, plasma osmolality decreases to about 10 mosm/kg below the non-pregnant norm due to a reduction in the plasma concentration of sodium and associated anions. There is a resetting of the osmostat in pregnancy with the osmotic thresholds for ADH release and thirst decreasing during the initial weeks of pregnancy. Osmoregulation may also be affected by changes in ADH metabolism, which are peculiar to pregnancy. The placenta produces vasopressinase which is capable of inactivating circulating ADH and can directly metabolize ADH *in situ*. Hence the placenta is thought to be responsible for at least 1/3 of ADH metabolism in pregnancy. The relationship between plasma ADH and plasma osmolality during pregnancy is shown in Fig. 11.3.

Renal tubular function in pregnancy

Some changes in plasma and urine biochemistry during pregnancy are summarized in Table 11.1.

Plasma *uric acid* concentrations decrease by 25–35% during early pregnancy due to increased uric acid excretion and clearance. As pregnancy progresses, excretion progressively falls and hence plasma uric acid levels gradually increase towards normal non-pregnant levels. In pregnancies complicated by pre-eclampsia (see below), plasma uric acid concentration is significantly elevated due to enhanced renal reabsorption of uric acid. Plasma uric acid levels above 0.35 mmol/L are associated with a significantly increased perinatal morbidity. Hence the uric acid level can be monitored to assess progress in pre-eclampsia.

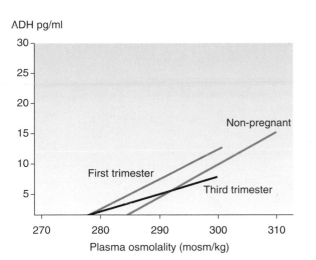

Fig. 11.3 Relationship between plasma levels of antidiuretic hormone (ADH) and plasma osmolality in non-pregnant subjects, and in the first and third trimesters of normal pregnancy.

Table 11.1 Changes in blood and urine biochemistry during pregnancy

Blood	Effect of pregnancy
Plasma uric acid	↓
Plasma sodium	↓
Plasma potassium	N – ↓
Plasma bicarbonate	↓
Arterial pCO₂	↓
Arterial pH	↑
Urine	
Glucose excretion	↑
Amino acid excretion	↑
Calcium excretion	↑
Magnesium excretion	↑
Citrate excretion	↑

Glucose excretion is commonly increased in normal pregnancy, with excretory rates normalizing to zero within a week of delivery. *Aminoaciduria* similarly may be observed in pregnancy. Up to 2 g of amino acid may be excreted daily which generally has few clinical consequences. It is considered that the increased GFR increases the filtered load of glucose and amino acids, and the proximal tubules do not have the capacity to increase their reabsorptive rates to match. Hence the glycosuria observed in a proportion of pregnant women does not in itself suggest a diagnosis of diabetes mellitus.

Acid base regulation is altered in pregnancy. The blood concentration of hydrogen ions decreases by 2–4 mmol/L in early pregnancy and this change is sustained until delivery. Blood concentrations of bicarbonate similarly fall by about 4 mmol/L such that a normal plasma bicarbonate level in pregnancy is between 18 and 22 mmol/L. Thus

the average arterial pH in pregnancy is 7.44 compared to 7.40 in the non-pregnant individual. The mild alkalosis is primarily respiratory in origin as progesterone induces an increase in respiratory rate which reduces the arterial pCO₂ from an average value of 40 mm Hg to approximately 32 mm Hg during pregnancy.

The regulation of *potassium* excretion by the kidney is significantly altered in pregnancy. It would be expected that the high levels of aldosterone and other mineralocorticoids during pregnancy, as well as lower blood concentrations of hydrogen, would lead to increased renal excretion of potassium. However, this is not observed and indeed there is a net retention of potassium in pregnancy, although plasma potassium concentration generally remains normal or even slightly decreased. The conservation of potassium has been ascribed to progesterone.

A net increase in urinary *calcium* excretion occurs in pregnancy, again attributed to the increase in filtered load of calcium which is not matched by a parallel increase in tubular calcium reabsorption. However, no increase in renal stone formation is seen in pregnancy due to parallel increases in urine flow rate and in urinary excretion of citrate and magnesium (known inhibitors of stone formation) and of acidic glycoproteins, including Tamm Horsfall protein, which inhibit calcium oxalate deposition.

Blood pressure and pregnancy

Blood pressure decreases early in normal pregnancy, with diastolic values typically 5–10 mm Hg below pre-pregnancy values by the 2nd trimester (see Fig. 11.4). In the third trimester, blood pressure generally returns towards normal, signifying a return of normal vasomotor tone. Since cardiac output increases, the drop in blood pressure reflects a marked decrease in peripheral vascular resistance, due in part to vasodilation in the uteroplacental bed. However, vasodilation also occurs in other organ systems such as the kidney and skin. Vasodilation occurs despite increases in systemic levels of renin and angiotensin II, signifying a loss of responsiveness to the pressor effects of angiotensin II. Conversely there is a normal pressor response to catecholamines in pregnancy. Increased production of prostaglandins (particularly by the pregnant uterus) and nitric oxide are considered to mediate the decrease in maternal vascular resistance observed in pregnancy.

Hypertension in pregnancy

Hypertension in pregnancy is diagnosed when the systolic blood pressure (SBP) is ≥140 mm Hg and/or diastolic BP is ≥90 mm Hg. Consistency of the readings should be documented with several measurements over a number of hours. Blood pressure is measured in the seated position with the feet supported, using an appropriately sized cuff. Approximately 10% of primigravidae will develop

Hypertension in pregnancy: 1

Denise Gill, a 36-year-old primigravid school teacher, presented for her first antenatal visit at 9 weeks gestation. An ultrasound, done by her GP the previous week, demonstrated a dizygotic twin pregnancy. She had been well in the past but when questioned, admitted that on being checked for prior prescriptions for the oral contraceptive pill, her blood pressure was generally 'on the high side'. However, no treatment had been suggested. Her younger sister had recently developed pre-eclampsia in her first pregnancy necessitating delivery at 36 weeks. Her mother had no history of pregnancy-related illness, but her grandmother had 'toxaemia' requiring bed rest for 6 weeks prior to the birth of her mother. She was a non-smoker, drank little alcohol, had recently commenced 'pregnancy' vitamins, but otherwise took no regular medications.

On examination, her body mass index was $30\,kg/m^2$. Her blood pressure was 140/90 mm Hg on repeated measurements, using a large cuff in both right and left arms. Examination of the optic fundi revealed minor arteriovenous nipping but no other abnormalities. Urinalysis was negative.

Denise was provided with a sphygmomanometer and instructed how to measure her blood pressure at home, and to return in one month with records of twice-daily BP measurements. Baseline 'pregnancy' blood tests (full blood count, blood group, rubella, hepatitis, syphilis and HIV serology) and an MSU had already been taken by her GP and were all normal. Additional bloods were requested to assess her renal function, liver function and uric acid.

Denise was concerned about the implications of having 'borderline' hypertension in pregnancy, the potential risks to both her and her unborn baby, and whether lifestyle modifications would help control her hypertension.

Fig. 11.4 Changes in blood pressure during normal pregnancy. PP, post-partum.

Box 11.2 Classification of hypertension in pregnancy (Society of Obstetric Medicine of Australia and New Zealand)

- Gestational hypertension
- Pre-eclampsia
- Chronic hypertension
  Essential
  Secondary
- Pre-eclampsia superimposed on chronic hypertension

gestational hypertension (see below) and 7% will develop pre-eclampsia. A small proportion of women will manifest signs and symptoms of hypertension or pre-eclampsia predominantly in the immediate post-partum period.

The Consensus Statement of the Society of Obstetric Medicine of Australia and New Zealand regarding the detection, investigation and management of hypertension in pregnancy classifies hypertension in pregnancy as shown in Box 11.2.

Gestational hypertension

Gestational hypertension is hypertension arising in pregnancy after 20 weeks gestation without any other feature of pre-eclampsia.

Pre-eclampsia

Pre-eclampsia is generally detected initially because of hypertension. However it is now recognized as a multi-system disorder in the mother with features shown in Fig. 11.5. Pre-eclampsia additionally has significant fetal manifestations and consequences, manifesting as intra-uterine growth retardation and rarely fetal death. A serious deterioration in the mother's condition is marked by the occurrence of a seizure, often accompanied by a decrease in level of consciousness. This turn of events is termed eclampsia.

Interesting facts

Eclampsia comes from the Greek word eklampsis, meaning a sudden flashing. It was introduced when it was believed that seizures in pregnancy occurred without any pre-existing disorder, and hence came 'like a flash of lightning'. It is now known that eclampsia always follows some degree of preceding pre-eclampsia, although the duration may be brief. Both pre-eclampsia and eclampsia used to be considered forms of 'toxaemia' of pregnancy.

The criteria for the diagnosis of pre-eclampsia are shown in Box 11.3. Note that oedema is not one of the diagnostic criteria of pre-eclampsia as it is often seen in otherwise normal pregnancy. Similarly an elevation

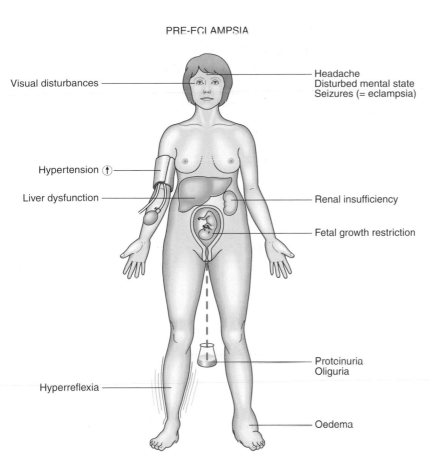

PRE-ECLAMPSIA

Visual disturbances

Headache
Disturbed mental state
Seizures (= eclampsia)

Hypertension (↑)

Liver dysfunction

Renal insufficiency

Fetal growth restriction

Proteinuria
Oliguria

Hyperreflexia

Oedema

Fig. 11.5 Clinical features of pre-eclampsia.

Box 11.3 Definition of pre-eclampsia

Hypertension arising after 20 weeks gestation plus the new onset of at least one of the following:

- Proteinuria (spot urine protein to creatinine ratio of ≥30 mg/mmol)
- Renal insufficiency (plasma creatinine greater than 0.09 mmol/L or oliguria)
- Liver disease (defined as raised transaminases)
- Neurological signs (hyperreflexia with clonus; headaches with hyperreflexia and/or visual disturbances; altered mental state)[1]
- Haematological disturbances (low platelet count, disseminated intravascular coagulation, haemolysis)
- Fetal growth restriction

[1]The occurrence of seizures defines the onset of eclampsia.

in plasma uric acid is not included in the criteria, but remains a useful marker, particularly to follow the course of an individual with pre-eclampsia.

Pre-eclampsia may rarely occur prior to 20 weeks gestation in patients with hydatidiform mole, multiple pregnancy, fetal triploidy and with prothrombotic disorders or renal disease. Other disorders may present with some of the features observed in pre-eclampsia: these include acute fatty liver of pregnancy, HELLP syndrome (haemolysis, elevated liver enzymes, low platelet count), anti-phospholipid syndrome, thrombotic thrombocytopaenia purpura and haemolytic uraemic syndrome. The differential diagnosis is made based on the constellation of clinical and laboratory findings.

Factors marking pregnant women at increased risk of pre-eclampsia are listed in Box 11.4. However, it should be noted that severe pre-eclampsia can occur, particularly in the primigravid individual, with no other risk factor. Additional features that alert the clinician to the possibility of developing pre-eclampsia include the failure of blood pressure to fall by mid pregnancy, and the *de novo* appearance of proteinuria in the second half of pregnancy.

Current views on the aetiology and pathogenesis of pre-eclampsia consider that the condition arises due to a combination of genetic and environmental factors resulting in abnormal placentation. Although there is a clear familial element in the development of the disease, the mode of inheritance remains elusive. Some evidence also suggests a paternal or fetal influence in the triggering of the condition, or alternatively a maternal–fetal genotype-by-genotype interaction. The incidence of pre-eclampsia is increased in women who live at high altitude and in areas of low socioeconomic status, suggesting as yet undefined environmental factors may additionally influence the development of pre-eclampsia.

Box 11.4 Risk factors for the development of pre-eclampsia

- Primigravida
- Multigravida pregnant by a different partner
- Maternal age greater than 40 years
- Prior pre-eclampsia in a pregnancy by the same partner
- Family history of pre-eclampsia
- Multiple pregnancy
- Obesity
- Renal disease
- Essential hypertension
- Diabetes
- Autoimmune disease, particularly systemic lupus erythematosus and the antiphospholipid syndrome
- Thrombophilia
- Severe alloimmunization

Pathologically, the maternal spiral arteries supplying blood to the fetoplacental unit fail to develop into sac-like flaccid vessels, retaining a muscular arteriole phenotype leading to decreased placental perfusion and placental ischaemia.

Recently it has been proposed that ischaemic placentas produce anti-angiogenic factors, such as a soluble receptor for vascular endothelial growth factor and placental growth factor called sFlt-1, which may be the link between disordered implantation and maternal symptoms of pre-eclampsia. Most of the maternal features of the condition (Fig. 11.5) are associated with vascular endothelial dysfunction and/or vasoconstriction in the various organ systems affected by the disease process, although much remains to be discovered of the precise mechanisms involved.

Chronic hypertension

Essential hypertension is defined as high blood pressure in those women already on antihypertensive drugs, or when systolic BP ≥140 mm Hg and/or diastolic BP ≥90 mm Hg pre-conception or in the first half of pregnancy with no underlying cause. *Secondary hypertension* is defined as in the non-pregnant population, i.e. hypertension associated with an underlying condition, particularly renal parenchymal, renovascular or endocrine disorders.

White coat hypertension, i.e. hypertension in the presence of a clinician but not observed in ambulatory or home BP assessments, is not considered to portend an adverse clinical outcome.

Pre-eclampsia superimposed on chronic hypertension

The presence of chronic hypertension is a risk factor for the development of pre-eclampsia. In patients with chronic hypertension, the development of proteinuria,

Case 11.2 Hypertension in pregnancy: 2

Initial treatment

Denise returned at 12 weeks gestation and remained feeling well. Her blood pressure readings had consistently been between 120/70 mm Hg and 140/90 mm Hg. Her plasma creatinine was 0.06 mmol/L, liver function tests normal and her plasma uric acid was 0.20 mmol/L. Her risk factors for developing pre-eclampsia complicating chronic hypertension were explained, i.e. twin pregnancy, obesity, pre-existing hypertension and her positive family history. She was advised to return to the clinic every 4 weeks, but to continue monitoring her blood pressure at home and advise if it was increasing to over 140/90 mm Hg.

At 28 weeks gestation she presented with worsening hypertension up to 150/100 mm Hg, but with no proteinuria. She was monitored in a day stay obstetric unit. Fetal movements and heart sounds were present and fetal growth was assessed as normal. Repeat blood tests were undertaken in conjunction with a routine 50 g oral glucose load, which was normal. Her plasma uric acid was 0.36 mmol/L, but other blood test results were normal. She was commenced on treatment with oxprenolol 80 mg bd and asked to return for review in one week.

Denise is now concerned that she has developed pre-eclampsia, and asks about the effect of medication on the fetus, the likelihood of premature delivery and whether she should stop work as it has been particularly stressful of late.

rapidly increasing blood pressure, right upper quadrant pain signifying liver involvement, or neurological symptoms should be considered highly suggestive of superimposed pre-eclampsia.

Management of hypertension in pregnancy

The management of hypertension in pregnancy needs to take into account both maternal and fetal factors. It should be noted that controlling the blood pressure does not in itself cure pre-eclampsia but it is indicated to avoid maternal cerebrovascular and cardiovascular complications.

Patients with gestational or chronic hypertension can usually be managed in the outpatient setting. Bed rest has not been shown to be of benefit in the treatment of hypertension in pregnancy. Obstetric units generally have individualized protocols for the use of oral antihypertensive agents during pregnancy. In general, shorter-acting, 'older' antihypertensive agents are used. These include the beta-blocker oxprenolol, centrally-acting agents alpha-methyldopa and clonidine, as well as others such as hydralazine, nifedipine, verapamil, labetolol, and prazosin. Longer acting beta-blockers, such as atenolol, are not recommended as they have been shown to be associated with impaired fetal growth. Angiotensin-converting enzyme inhibitors and angiotensin receptor blockers should not be prescribed during pregnancy since their use, particularly during the third trimester, has been linked with the development of fetal growth retardation, oligohydramnios, neonatal renal failure and death. Diuretics are also avoided since although oedema may be present, this is often in the setting of a reduction in effective plasma volume, and hence diuretics may exacerbate placental ischaemia.

Antihypertensive therapy is generally instituted when diastolic BP is greater than 90 mm Hg with the aim of keeping systolic BP between 120–140 mm Hg and diastolic BP 80–90 mm Hg. Antihypertensives utilized in pregnancy are also considered safe when breastfeeding. Hypertension in pregnancy does not generally preclude the opportunity to breastfeed.

Once a diagnosis of pre-eclampsia is made, the stage of gestation, the degree of maternal organ dysfunction, and fetal well-being all need to be considered in determining subsequent management. In addition to oral antihypertensive drugs, intravenous fluids may be indicated to correct central volume contraction, despite the presence of peripheral oedema. In patients with more severe hypertension (SBP >170 mm Hg or DBP >110 mm Hg) parenteral antihypertensive medication is required. Again local unit protocols should be developed for a consistent approach, but agents commonly used are IV or IM hydralazine or IV labetolol or diazoxide. In general, SBP should be lowered by 20–30 mm Hg and diastolic by 10–15 mm Hg to ensure maternal safety and to protect the fetal circulation. Continuous cardiotocography (CTG) monitoring of the fetal circulation should be undertaken when parenteral agents are used to lower critically elevated blood pressure in this setting.

If eclampsia has developed, the seizure should be terminated with the use of IV diazepam, prophylaxis against further convulsions provided with IV magnesium sulphate administration, the blood pressure controlled, and immediate delivery arranged. In impending eclampsia, when premonitory neurological signs are present, the use of IV magnesium sulphate can be considered. However, its use in this setting is controversial and delivery should be expedited.

In general, if either the mother or fetus is at risk of significant complications as a consequence of a hypertensive disease in pregnancy, delivery should be considered, particularly when the fetus is mature. General indications for delivery in this context are given in Box 11.5.

When delivery pre-term is indicated because of severe pre-eclampsia, particularly if fetal compromise is present, then caesarean section will generally be required, with arrangements made for resuscitation and support of the baby in a neonatal intensive care unit.

Follow-up of patients with hypertension in pregnancy

In patients with severe pre-eclampsia, maternal complications may develop for up to 5 days post-partum. Hence

---

Box 11.5 General indications for delivery in hypertensive disorders of pregnancy

- Pre-eclampsia occurring at term
- Accelerated hypertension uncontrollable on treatment
- Deteriorating renal or liver function
- Progressive thrombocytopenia
- Neurological complications suggesting imminent eclampsia
- Placental abruption
- Fetal compromise

Case 11.2 Hypertension in pregnancy: 3

Further treatment and outcome

Denise was followed up regularly, her oxprenolol increased to maximal doses and hydralazine added to her treatment over the next 8 weeks. At 36 weeks gestation she presented complaining of headache and swollen ankles. Examination showed her BP to be 170/110 mm Hg, she had moderate oedema, 3+ proteinuria and two beats of ankle clonus. A CTG of both fetuses showed a normal pattern.

She was given 5 mg hydralazine intravenously which brought her blood pressure down to 160/100 mm Hg, but over the next 90 minutes it again increased to 175/105 mm Hg. Her blood tests showed a platelet count of 162×10^9/L (previously 250×10^9/L), uric acid 0.46 mmol/L, AST 70 IU/L, with other blood tests normal. Her urine protein to creatinine ratio was 424 mg/mmol. Caesarean section was arranged as had been planned, as one twin had consistently been in a breech position. Epidural anaesthesia resulted in a fall in blood pressure to 130/80 mm Hg, and an uneventful caesarian delivery occurred. Following delivery her blood pressure remained well controlled on oral medication and her drug treatment was progressively weaned. She was advised to follow up her blood pressure with her general practitioner and to return for review in 3 months.

She was concerned about her ability to breast feed and, although not an immediate priority, about her risks in a future pregnancy.

---

vigilance in monitoring is required. As blood pressure settles, antihypertensives may be withdrawn. However, immediately after delivery there may be a reduction in blood pressure due to blood loss and the use of epidural anaesthesia, but hypertension may later reappear. Review is undertaken 3 months post-partum to ensure that blood pressure has settled and urinalysis is normal, and if laboratory tests have not normalized post delivery, these should be reassessed. Investigations for an underlying thrombophilic state, renal disease or autoimmune disease

Introduction

Loin pain may arise because of pathology in the nerves radiating from the spinal cord, vertebral column, paraspinal and lumbar muscles, and retroperitoneal organs such as kidneys, abdominal aorta and pancreas. The simultaneous presence of haematuria strongly suggests that the loin pain is caused by pathology in the kidneys or ureters. If loin pain and/or haematuria are present, then it is necessary to consider whether urinary tract obstruction is also present. The following case history describes a patient with a renal calculus (stone) causing loin pain, haematuria and urinary obstruction. See 12.1: 1.

Differential diagnosis of loin pain and haematuria

Any back or retroperitoneal structure may give rise to back pain (Box 12.1). Pain arising from spasm of a tubular or hollow organ, such as the ureter, is referred to as colic. The severity and radiation of this patient's pain were typical of renal colic, although pain of a similar distribution could occur because of compression or involvement of a nerve root. The extension of the pain into his right groin and inner right thigh is explained by movement of the pathology down the ureter (Fig. 12.1). Kidney pain arises because of rapid stretching or inflammation of the kidney capsule, whereas pain arising from the renal pelvis

or ureter is caused by distension and excessive peristaltic contractions.

Macroscopic haematuria may arise from lesions anywhere within the urinary system, including the kidney itself, the renal pelvis, ureter, bladder and urethra. As few as 5×10^6 red cells per millilitre (1 microlitre of blood per millilitre of urine) can be detected visually as red-coloured urine.

Macroscopic haematuria needs to be distinguished from the following:

- Red discolouration of urine caused by certain dyes and occasional drugs (e.g. rifampicin).

- The presence of haem pigment in the case of intravascular haemolysis (haemoglobin from red blood cell lysis) or rhabdomyolysis (myoglobin from muscle breakdown).

- Bleeding outside the urinary tract (e.g. perineum or vagina).

The relationship of the blood to urine helps to distinguish bleeding involving the bladder or above

Box 12.1 Principal sites of pathology leading to loin pain

Spinal nerve roots
Vertebral column
Paraspinal and lumbar muscles
Kidneys
Renal pelvis/ureters
Abdominal aorta
Pancreas

Case 12.1 Urinary tract obstruction and stones: 1

Loin pain and haematuria

Kevin Whiteside is a 63-year-old man who presented to the Casualty department of his local hospital with a 6h history of right-sided pain and smoky (reddish-grey) urine. The loin pain was situated at the level of the first three lumbar vertebrae and radiated around the right side of his abdomen. After several hours it radiated further into his right testis and the upper medial aspect of his right thigh. The pain was constant and very severe. His right kidney was ballottable and very tender. (Ballottement refers to the rebound felt by the hand placed over the middle–upper quadrant of the abdomen when the fingers of the other hand tap upwards in the loin to displace the kidney.) He was afebrile, sweating and pale. His blood pressure and the remainder of his physical examination were normal. Urinalysis was strongly positive for blood.

The main features in this patient's history were the presence of severe loin pain and macroscopic haematuria. The haematuria suggested strongly that the pain originated in the urinary tract rather than other potential sites.

Fig. 12.1 Site of renal colic. Renal colic typically radiates from the loin around to the lower quadrant of the abdomen and the upper medial thigh on the same side.

Table 12.1 Differential diagnosis of red urine

	With loin pain	Uniform discoloration of urine	Haem pigment on dipstick	Red blood cells in urine	Casts and protein in urine	Predominantly dysmorphic red blood cells
Foods and dyes (e.g. beetroot)	–	+	–	–	–	–
Drugs (e.g. rifampicin)	–	+	–	–	–	–
Pigmenturia (haemolysis or rhabdomyolysis)	–	+	+	–	–	–
Non-urological bleeding	–	–	+	+	–	–
Urethral bleeding	–	–	+	+	–	–
Renal, ureteric or bladder tumours	–*	+	+	+	–	–
Calculi or infection	+	+	+	+	–	–
Renal parenchymal lesion (glomerulonephritis or interstitial nephritis)	±	+	+	+	+	+

*Ureteric and bladder tumours may cause pain because of obstruction.

(uniform discoloration of urine) from that arising from the urethra (blood separate or mixed with urine).

Haematuria arising from the kidney parenchyma (glomeruli or interstitium) tends to be accompanied by proteinuria and casts, whereas bleeding arising from renal tumours or from lesions in the renal pelvis or below may be isolated or (particularly with infection) associated with pyuria (white blood cells in the urine). Moreover, most red blood cells arising from kidney parenchymal lesions have an abnormal morphology (best appreciated by phase contrast microscopy), whereas those from renal tumours or more distal lesions have a normal biconcave appearance (Table 12.1). Red cells may also be damaged by urine of high osmolality (which causes cell shrinkage) or low osmolality (causes cell swelling and haemolysis). With brisk bleeding there may be frank blood with little urine.

Macroscopic haematuria arising from tumours tends to be painless, whereas that arising from calculi or infection is usually associated with pain. Occasionally, crystals (microcalculi) can cause pain and macroscopic haematuria. Renal calculi are discussed in more detail later in this chapter and urological tumours in Chapter 13.

See 12.1: 2.

Imaging of the urinary tract

As outlined in Chapter 1 (in the context of urinary tract infection), there are multiple investigations from which to choose to image the urinary tract. These are summarized in Table 12.2. Each has particular attributes so the choice depends on the suspected diagnosis and the question to be answered.

In the investigation of loin pain and macroscopic haematuria, adequate information can usually be obtained from simple investigations. As 90% of renal calculi are radio-opaque, the plain abdominal X-ray is a useful first test (see Fig. 12.2). Ultrasonography is cheap and non-invasive, and provides useful information about renal size, renal mass lesions (in particular cysts), and renal pelvic and ureteric dilatation (see Fig. 12.3). Increasingly, an abdominal CT scan is performed relatively early in the investigation of possible abnormalities of the urinary tract and to define the site and cause of urinary tract obstruction (see Fig. 12.4).

Interesting facts

Ultrasonography is useful for demonstrating hydronephrosis and hydroureter. The kidney pelvis and ureter may appear dilated when the bladder is full of urine, so in that case it is sometimes necessary to repeat the examination after the bladder has been emptied.

Pathophysiology of urinary tract obstruction

The presence of renal pelvic dilatation (hydronephrosis) on the current patient's ultrasound scan indicates a partial or complete obstruction to urinary flow; there was no hydroureter, consistent with the obstruction being caused by the calculus at the level of the pelviureteric junction. Stones of 1cm or greater diameter are unlikely to pass beyond this level spontaneously. As with any hollow organ, obstruction could be due to an extrinsic, intramural or luminal lesion. Common causes of urinary tract obstruction are shown in Fig. 12.5.

The patient's age and gender and clinical setting often allow accurate prediction of the cause of obstruction. For example, in an elderly male obstruction is commonly due to prostatic enlargement, whereas in an elderly female it might be due to a gynaecological tumour. Obstruction may

Case 12.1 Urinary tract obstruction and stones: 2

Obstruction

As the pain was typical of renal colic, Kevin was suspected of having a renal calculus. A plain abdominal X-ray was arranged; this demonstrated a large radio-opaque lesion lying to the right of the L2/L3 vertebrae (Fig. 12.2). An abdominal ultrasound demonstrated dilatation of the right renal pelvis (hydronephrosis) above a hyperechogenic, shadowing lesion (renal calculus) with normal thickness and echogenicity of the right kidney (Fig. 12.3).

The imaging of the patient's renal tract demonstrated a renal calculus causing blockage of urinary flow. These findings give rise to the following questions:

1. What are the different modalities for imaging the urinary tract? Which are the best for a patient with a suspected renal calculus?
2. Why do renal calculi occur?
3. What are the consequences of urinary tract obstruction caused by a renal calculus?

Each of these questions will be answered below.

Fig. 12.2 Plain abdominal X-ray of the current patient showing a radio-opaque calculus near the second and third lumbar vertebrae on the right.

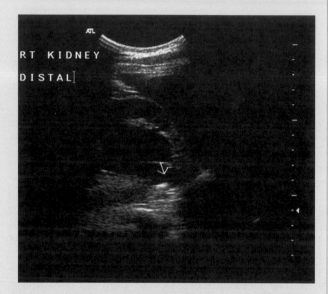

Fig. 12.3 Ultrasound scan of the right kidney of the current patient showing dilatation of the renal pelvis and an echogenic lesion (arrowed) at the pelviureteric junction, associated with an acoustic shadow beneath it. The denser an object is in relation to water the brighter it appears on ultrasound (echogenic). Note how the contents of the renal pelvis (urine) appear black, that is, non-echogenic.

be bilateral, in particular with lesions of the bladder or urethra, when it poses a particular risk of causing renal failure.

As a result of urinary flow obstruction, resting intraluminal pressure rises (from 1 up to 80 mm Hg) and leads to proximal functional and structural changes. Ureteral peristalsis increases in frequency and amplitude initially. The ureter and renal pelvis dilate (Fig. 12.6) and, with persistent obstruction, peristalsis diminishes and becomes disorganized, and intraluminal pressure falls.

The pressure effects are transmitted to the kidney and lead to a range of structural and functional changes (Box 12.2). As might be predicted, distal tubular function becomes compromised with impairment of the following:

- water and sodium reabsorption
- urinary concentration
- acid and potassium secretion.

After an initial phase of compensatory vasodilatation, glomerular filtration rate (GFR) and renal blood flow fall because of a combination of the back-pressure effects and release of locally active vasoconstrictor hormones (in particular thromboxane A_2 and angiotensin II), which alter intrarenal haemodynamics (Fig. 12.7).

Table 12.2 Imaging of the urinary tract

Test	Particularly useful for:	Cost
Plain abdominal X-ray	Radio-opaque calculi	+
Plain renal tomogram	Renal size and outline	+
Intravenous pyelogram*	Renal size, outline and function (nephrogram)	++
	Renal pelvis, ureter and bladder (excretory phase)	
Retrograde pyelogram*	Bladder visualization by cystoscopy**, ureter and renal pelvis	++++
Antegrade pyelogram*	Obstructed renal pelvis and ureter	+++
Ultrasonography	Renal cysts, size and pelvis	++
Dynamic isotope scan†	Renal blood flow, differential function, and outflow	++
Static isotope scan†	Renal size and scars	++
CT scan (+/− contrast)	Renal mass lesions, non-radio-opaque calculi	++++
Spiral CT	Renal artery anatomy	
Magnetic resonance imaging	Renal mass lesions	++++
Magnetic resonance angiography	Renal arterial flow	

*A pyelogram is an X-ray image of the renal pelvis.

**Cystoscopy is an endoscopic examination of the bladder performed prior to contrast injection up the ureters.

†'Dynamic' isotopes (e.g. **DTPA**) are filtered and excreted by the kidney, whereas 'static' isotopes (e.g. **DMSA**) are taken up by renal cells.

Fig. 12.4 A, Pelvic CT scan showing stone fragment in lower right ureter (arrow). B, Abdominal CT scan showing dilated right renal pelvis (arrow) above an obstructing calculus.

These functional changes may be reversible with relief of acute obstruction, or partially reversible or irreversible with prolonged obstruction, leading to renal scarring. Characteristically, with the relief of obstruction and therefore the passage of urine, the distal functional defects may become manifest clinically. This is called postobstructive diuresis, caused by an osmotic and physiological diuresis due to excretion of retained water, sodium and urea.

A persistent defect in collecting duct function involving impaired aquaporin 2-mediated water reabsorption (a form of nephrogenic diabetes insipidus; see Chapter 3) contributes to postobstructive diuresis. Renal scarring occurs over a period of weeks because of the effects of pressure and the release of chemoattractant and fibrogenic cytokines, such as osteopontin and monocyte chemoattractant protein 1, and transforming growth factor β, respectively.

(A) **Obstruction can be intraluminal, intramural, extrinsic**

Extrinsic
– trauma
– tumour
– inflammation
– infection
– haemorrhage
– fibrosis

Intramural
– transitional cell cancer
– fibrosis
– inflammation
– infection

Intraluminal
– calculus
– blood clot
– renal papilla

Congenital pelviureteric
junction obstruction

Retroperitoneal fibrosis,
tumours, haemorrhage

Cancer of
– ovary
– cervix
– uterus

'Functional'— vesicoureteric reflux
— neurogenic bladder

Bladder cancer

Prostatic hypertrophy
or cancer
Urethral stricture or valve

(B) **Common causes of obstruction**

Fig. 12.5 Sites and causes of urinary obstruction.

Hydronephrosis

Thinned, scarred
renal cortex
(chronic)

Unobstructed

Hydroureter
(above the level
of obstruction)

Fig. 12.6 Structural consequences of urinary tract obstruction.

With unilateral, slowly progressive and/or partial obstruction, the symptoms and clinical and laboratory signs of obstruction may not be obvious.

Renal calculi

Renal calculi (stones) are a common cause of loin pain, haematuria and urinary tract obstruction. Some 90% of calculi are radio-opaque and so may be detected by plain radiography, as with the current patient.

Common types of renal calculi are listed in Table 12.3. An illustration of the physical characteristics of specific types of stone is given in Fig. 12.8. Urinary stasis, caused by poor urine output or obstruction, is an important pathogenic factor in the formation of most stones. Other factors relevant in particular cases include altered urinary pH, low

Box 12.2 Functional consequences of urinary tract obstruction

Reduced glomerular filtration rate
Reduced renal blood flow (after an initial rise)
Impaired renal concentrating ability
Impaired distal tubular function
    Nephrogenic diabetes insipidus
    Renal salt wasting
    Renal tubular acidosis
    Impaired potassium secretion
Postobstructive diuresis

concentration of naturally occurring stone inhibitors (e.g. citrate), infection (especially with microorganisms that split urea to form ammonia), and excess urinary excretion of the substances which form stones owing to excess dietary intake, systemic overproduction or release, and/ or reduced renal reabsorption.

The current patient's calculus was causing obstruction of urinary flow, and was too large to pass to the bladder spontaneously. This raises the question of what would happen if the obstruction were not relieved, and

Pathophysiology of changes in —

	Intraluminal pressure	RBF	GFR
Phase A	↑ ...due to : Obstruction ↑ Peristalsis	↑ ...due to : Vasodilatation — prostacyclin — prostaglandin E_2	↓ ...due to : ↑ Intratubular pressure
Phase B	↓ ...due to : Disorganized peristalsis Dilation of tubules and ureter	↓ ...due to : Vasoconstriction — angiotensin II — thromboxane A_2	↓ ...due to : — continuing obstruction — vasoconstriction

Fig. 12.7 Functional consequences of acute urinary tract obstruction.

Table 12.3 Renal calculi

Composition	Percentage	Radio-opaque	Appearance	Crystal shape	Pathogenesis
Calcium oxalate	60	+++	Small, smooth or spiky	'Back of envelope' or dumb-bell	Hyperparathyroidism, hypercalciuria, hypocitraturia, hyperoxaluria, hyperuricosuria
Calcium phosphate	20	+++	Slightly larger, more friable	Elongated	High urine pH due to distal renal tubular acidosis
Uric acid	<10	−	May be large	Rhomboidal	Low urine pH, hyperuricosuria
Struvite ($MgNH_4PO_4$)	<10	++	Staghorn	'Coffin lid'	Infection with urease-producing microorganisms, causing high urine pH
Cystine	<5	+	Pale yellow, may be large	Hexagonal	Cystinuria

how should the stone be treated. These issues will be addressed in the last section of this chapter.

See 12.1: 3.

Interesting facts

Some kidney stones particularly those that fill the renal pelvis (staghorn calculus) can be quite large; these include stones which are composed mainly of uric acid, struvite or cystine. The largest kidney stone is reported to have weighed 1.36 kg!

Principles of treatment

With urinary tract obstruction, the main principle of treatment is to relieve the obstruction to prevent functional and structural damage to the kidney (Table 12.4). If left untreated for a period of weeks, this damage becomes irreversible. However, with superadded urinary infection the patient may become septicaemic and develop pyonephrosis (an infected obstructed kidney) with rapid renal destruction: these conditions require emergency treatment. Stones

(A)   (B)   (C)

Fig. 12.8 Macroscopic appearance of renal calculi. A, Staghorn calculus (forming a cast of the calyces and renal pelvis); B, spiculated (spiked) stones of calcium oxalate ('mulberry' stones or 'jackstones'); C, lamellated (layered) bladder stones, mainly of uric acid. Specimens courtesy of the Department of Urology, Concord Hospital.

Case 12.1 Urinary tract obstruction and stones: 3

Infection and treatment

Over the next 24h the patient became febrile (39°C), with **rigors** and an increase in left loin pain. The peripheral white cell count rose to *15.0 × 10⁹/L with a predominant neutrophilia. It was felt that infection had developed proximal to the obstructing stone.

The patient was started on intravenous antibiotics and, on the same day, was taken to the operating theatre. Here the stone was manipulated by ureteric instrumentation back into the renal pelvis and a ureteric stent placed to relieve the obstruction. (A stent is a narrow tube which is placed within the ureter to maintain its patency.) Between 50 and 100mL of purulent fluid passed through the ureter when the stent was placed. The patient improved over the next few days.

Four weeks later he underwent extracorporeal lithotripsy (shattering of a calculus using external shock waves) and subsequently passed a number of stone fragments (Fig. 12.9). These were analysed and shown to consist predominantly of calcium and oxalate.

With stasis of urinary flow, microorganisms are not flushed out and can multiply. The addition of infection to the patient's clinical picture turned this into a condition which required emergency treatment.

*Values outside the normal range; see Appendix.

Fig. 12.9 Plain abdominal X-ray showing stone fragments after extracorporeal lithotripsy of the stone shown in Fig. 12.2.

Table 12.4 Principles of treatment of renal calculi

Emergency	Narcotic analgesics for pain relief
	Long-acting alpha-blocking and calcium-blocking drugs to relieve ureteric spasm and promote stone passage
	Correction of fluid and electrolyte disturbances
	Intravenous antibiotics for systemic or intrarenal infection
	Relief of obstruction to treat infection and preserve renal function
Remove calculus	Endoluminal procedure, lithotripsy, or open operation
Determine pathogenesis	Stone analysis
	Fluid intake and dietary history
	Family history for genetic factors
	Serum and urinary 'metabolic screen'
Prevent further calculi	Increased fluid intake (e.g. 2.5–3 L/day)
	Modification of diet
	Specific treatment of metabolic abnormality

less than 1 cm in diameter may pass spontaneously, whereas larger stones require surgical intervention. Depending on their size, position and composition they may be treated with a combination of lithotripsy (to fracture the stone into fragments), endoluminal extraction (from within the urinary tract lumen) or open surgical removal.

Where possible, the pathogenesis of stone formation in a particular patient should be determined to guide appropriate treatment measures to prevent further stone formation. Pathogenesis can usually be inferred from a dietary history, history of fluid intake, information about familial occurrence, urinary culture, and a 'metabolic screen' of plasma and urine. The main components of the metabolic screen are determined by the usual or expected composition of the stone (see Table 12.3), and include plasma calcium and uric acid, urinary pH, calcium, uric acid, oxalate, citrate and, in some cases, cystine.

Interesting facts

It used to be thought that reducing dietary calcium intake might reduce the incidence of kidney stones. However, a large epidemiological study showed that dietary calcium restriction was actually associated with increased stone formation! This probably occurred because there would be less intestinal calcium to bind oxalate, leading to greater absorption of oxalate across the bowel and therefore increased urinary excretion of oxalate. Other changes in diet may have unrecognized effects on stone risk. For example, increased dietary fructose increases the risk of stone formation.

RENAL MASSES AND URINARY TRACT TUMOURS

13

Chapter objectives

After studying this chapter you should be able to:

1. Give the differential diagnosis of a renal mass.

2. List some risk factors for the development of renal cell carcinoma.

3. Describe the common presenting features of renal cell carcinoma.

4. Outline the principles of management of renal cell carcinoma.

5. List some risk factors for the development of bladder cancer.

6. Describe the common presenting features of bladder cancer.

7. Outline the principles of management of bladder cancer.

Introduction

Many drugs are excreted by the kidney through glomerular filtration, tubular secretion or a combination of these processes. Conjugated metabolites produced by the liver are also excreted by the kidney. Reduced renal clearances in patients with kidney disease may result in accumulation of drugs and their metabolites, with increased risk of toxicity. Renal dysfunction may also affect the distribution of the drug in the body by altering total body water, or the metabolism or protein-binding of the drug, which in turn may modify its therapeutic and adverse effects.

In addition to the effect of pre-existing renal dysfunction on drug excretion and metabolism, many drugs may themselves directly influence renal function through:

- Effects on volume status or renal haemodynamics that may alter the glomerular filtration rate (GFR).

- Accumulation of the drug or its metabolites causing direct toxicity to the kidney.

Mechanisms to 'protect' the kidney from nephrotoxic insults and to maintain cellular integrity exist, but these are likely to be impaired in the presence of chronic kidney disease, which further predisposes to drug nephrotoxicity. The list of potential agents contributing to acute kidney injury is extensive, and includes use of traditional medicines in some geographical areas. Hence a careful history should be undertaken with respect to both prescribed and complementary medicines in the investigation of an abrupt decrease in renal function.

This chapter will discuss the factors and mechanisms influencing drug excretion by the kidneys in patients with both normal and abnormal renal function in Part A. In Part B, the physiological and cellular basis for drug-induced nephropathies will be considered.

Effect of renal impairment on drug excretion

Case 14.1 Drugs and the kidney: 1

Too much digoxin?

Mrs Beverley Johnson is a 71-year-old woman who has been under treatment from her general practitioner for heart failure for several years. She has underlying ischaemic heart disease and suffered an acute myocardial infarction affecting the anterior wall of the left ventricle at the age of 68. Since that time, she has been treated with an angiotensin-converting enzyme (ACE) inhibitor (lisinopril 5 mg daily) and a diuretic (furosemide [frusemide] 40 mg twice daily).

Recently Mrs Johnson's condition deteriorated, with increased shortness of breath and fatigue. After admission to the local hospital's Emergency department, she was found to have developed **atrial fibrillation** and was started on digoxin 0.25 mg daily. Ten days after returning home from this admission, she called her GP to visit her because she had been experiencing increasing nausea with three episodes of vomiting since her discharge.

On examination, Mrs Johnson looks pale and uncomfortable, but is haemodynamically stable (blood pressure 130/80, pulse 86 beats/min, still in atrial fibrillation). She appears a little dry, and weighs 56 kg (usual weight 57–58 kg). The doctor checks his records, which reveal that Mrs Johnson's biochemistry (at the time of her recent admission) showed normal electrolytes, but slightly increased plasma concentrations of urea (*9.5 mmol/L) and creatinine (*0.14 mmol/L), reflecting some renal impairment presumed to be caused by vascular disease and poor cardiac output.

The doctor now suspects that digoxin toxicity has developed, and takes blood for a serum digoxin level as well as electrolytes and renal function. He advises her to stop taking the digoxin until he gets the results.

This case raises the following questions:

1. How is the kidney involved in the metabolism and excretion of drugs?
2. What characteristics of a drug are likely to predict whether the kidney has a primary role in determining its plasma concentration?
3. What patient characteristics influence the metabolism and excretion of a drug under normal circumstances?
4. How and when should drug dosing be modified in the presence of renal impairment?

Before we consider the specifics of Mrs Johnson's clinical problem, it is useful to consider the general principles involved in the normal metabolism and excretion of a drug that will influence its prescription.

*Values outside the normal range; see Appendix.

Principles of drug dosing

The dosage of a drug and the frequency with which it is given requires an understanding of both its pharmacodynamics and pharmacokinetics. Pharmacodynamics refers to the relationship between drug dose, plasma concentration and the effect of the drug. Pharmacokinetics describes the parameters of absorption, distribution and excretion of the drug: these factors determine the dose that should be administered and the dosage interval required to maximize effectiveness of the drug and minimize side effects. Many patient-related factors will influence the pharmacodynamics and pharmacokinetics, and this should be reflected in both the dosage and timing of drug administration.

An important pharmacodynamic concept is that the response to a drug is related to its concentration, either in plasma or in tissue. The classic relationship between dose and effect is demonstrated in Fig. 14.1A. It is clear from this relationship that a minimal concentration of drug is necessary to achieve a desired effect and that once a certain level of drug is reached no further therapeutic effect is gained. However, if higher concentrations of drug are obtained then toxicity may ensue. The overlap between toxic and beneficial effects is referred to as the therapeutic index. For some drugs there is a large difference between the drug levels at which maximum efficacy is achieved and toxicity develops (Fig. 14.1B). In these circumstances, dosage modification is not generally needed in renal failure, even if the drug accumulates to high levels (e.g. penicillin). However, other drugs have a narrow therapeutic index, which means that toxicity occurs at a level close to the maximal efficacy (Fig. 14.1C). It is in these circumstances that blood levels of the drug, generally taken just before the next planned dose, are most useful to ensure that efficacy is maintained and the risk of toxicity minimized. This is the case, for example, with digoxin.

Altered pharmacokinetics in renal disease

As described above, pharmacokinetic factors determine the plasma concentration achieved after a drug is administered. These factors include the absorption of the drug, its distribution in body fluids and tissue, and its excretion. All of these steps may be altered during renal disease, although the greatest effect is on excretion.

Gastrointestinal absorption

The amount of drug absorbed from the gastrointestinal tract largely depends on the characteristics of the drug rather than patient-related factors. However, in patients with renal impairment, the absorption of drugs from the gastrointestinal tract may be reduced because of gastric stasis, reduced gastric acidity and concurrent treatment with phosphate-binding drugs which will also bind numerous medications (e.g. aspirin, ciprofloxacin).

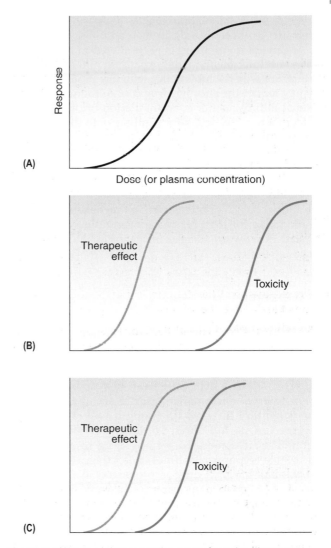

Fig. 14.1 Theoretical dose–response curves for a drug (response on y axis as percentage of maximum effect, dose on x axis as log drug concentration). (A) Basic dose–response relationship; (B) dose–response relationship for the therapeutic effect and the toxic effect of a particular drug (no overlap, i.e. wide therapeutic index); (C) dose–response relationship for the therapeutic and toxic effects of another drug (with overlap, i.e. narrow therapeutic index).

Drug distribution

The volume of distribution (V_d) of a drug is defined as the volume of fluid that the drug would need to be distributed in to produce the measured plasma concentration. It is calculated as follows:

$$V_d = \frac{\text{dose of drug administered}}{\text{plasma concentration}}$$

The volume of distribution for a drug exclusively confined to the plasma approximates the plasma volume. This is likely to be the case for drugs which are very highly protein-bound. If a drug is very water-soluble, then the volume of distribution approximates body water (approximately 60% of body weight in men and 55% in women). The volume of distribution may be altered in renal failure because of fluid retention and expansion of the circulating volume. For water-soluble drugs with low protein-binding, this may reduce the effective drug concentration.

Renal failure results in accumulation of organic acids that compete with drugs for binding onto albumin and other plasma proteins. As serum albumin may be low in renal failure, an increased proportion of free drug may be available. However, the changes in protein binding rarely require a change in the loading dose of drugs, nor in the interpretation of steady state plasma drug levels, with the exception of phenytoin. In this instance the therapeutic range for total plasma concentration needs to be adjusted downward to take into account increased free drug availability.

Renal excretion

The excretion of a drug (and its clearance) is related to the volume of distribution of the drug and its half-life ($t_{1/2}$), which is the time for its plasma concentration to halve after absorption and distribution of the drug are complete. The $t_{1/2}$ of a drug may help in determining dosage interval and predicting drug accumulation. It is often important to know how long it will take before a drug reaches its full effect, i.e. its steady state concentration. The time required for any drug to achieve this steady state is four to five times its $t_{1/2}$ (Fig. 14.2A).

If the half-life of a drug is prolonged in renal failure because of a reduction in clearance, then a widening of the dosage interval is required, and the time to reach steady state may be prolonged (Fig. 14.2B). This has implications for drugs such as digoxin, which normally has a $t_{1/2}$ of 36h, and thus steady state is reached after 1 week. However, in renal failure the $t_{1/2}$ is prolonged, and steady state may not be reached for several weeks. A corollary of this is that, where the dosing interval is not altered, administration of the usual dose of the drug will rapidly lead to accumulation of high serum concentrations (Fig. 14.2C). This may have serious clinical consequences for drugs such as digoxin, which have a narrow therapeutic index, and both the effective dose and toxicity correlate closely with the steady state plasma concentration.

The renal excretion of a drug is determined by filtration and the net effect of tubular secretion and reabsorption.

The filtration of a drug into the urine depends largely on its molecular weight and the degree to which it is protein-bound. In general, filtration is increased with a lower molecular weight and a lesser degree of protein binding. Once filtered, lipid-soluble drugs may be passively reabsorbed from the tubular fluid down a concentration gradient to the plasma. Water-soluble drugs may be 'trapped' in the tubular fluid and excreted if no specific reabsorptive mechanism exists.

Some drugs undergo active secretion into the urine by facilitated (carrier-mediated) transport mechanisms

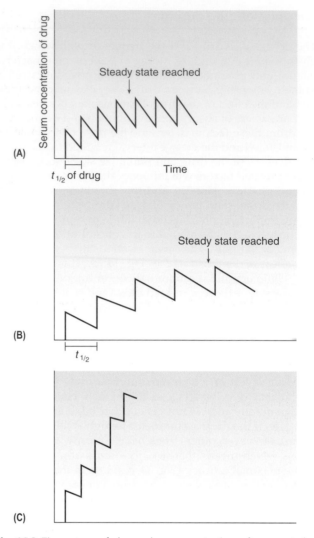

Fig. 14.2 Time course of plasma drug concentrations after repeated oral administration of the same dose at constant time intervals. (A) Drug administered at interval corresponding to its half-life of elimination ($t_{1/2}$); steady state reached in approximately five half-lives. (B) Same drug with prolonged half-life caused by reduced drug excretion in renal failure; when dose is given every (new) half-life, the time to steady state is greatly prolonged; (C) same drug given in renal failure at interval corresponding to half-life in normal renal function, resulting in rapid accumulation of drug to excessively high levels.

that normally transport organic acids or bases across the proximal tubular wall. The basic cellular mechanisms involved in this secretory process are illustrated in Fig. 14.3. It has been established that, for organic acids (including many anionic drugs), the initial step in secretion is the uptake of the anion into the cell across the basolateral membrane by cotransport with sodium, which enters the cell down its electrochemical gradient (generated by the action of the basolateral Na,K-ATPase). The anion then reaches a relatively high intracellular concentration and leaves the cell down its concentration gradient into the lumen, exchanging via a countertransport carrier with another anion such as chloride. The secretory

Fig. 14.3 Schematic of proximal tubular cell showing mechanism for transepithelial secretion of an organic acid (e.g. anionic drug).

Table 14.1 Drugs which are actively secreted by the proximal tubule

Organic acids	*Organic bases*
Penicillins	Amiloride
Cephalosporins	Quinidine
Sulphonamides	Tetracycline
Furosemide (frusemide)	
Thiazides	
Salicylates	
Probenicid	

mechanism for organic bases and cationic drugs is less well defined, but probably involves a primary secretory step across the apical cell membrane, with secondary increase in uptake across the basolateral membrane. A representative list of drugs undergoing secretion by one or other of these pathways is given in Table 14.1.

Drugs undergoing transport across the tubular epithelium may be affected by the pH of the tubular fluid. This is because the charged form of the drug (an organic acid in a high luminal pH environment or an organic base in a low luminal pH environment) is more water-soluble, favouring excretion (Fig. 14.4). Excretion of acidic drugs is therefore increased by raising the urinary pH, and the excretion of basic drugs is favoured by the excretion of an acidic urine. This may be important when facilitating drug excretion following overdosage, e.g. alkalinization of the urine with bicarbonate infusion to enhance aspirin excretion.

Finally, some drugs prevent the tubular secretion of other drugs by competing for binding to common transporters in the proximal tubule. This may be used therapeutically to enhance the desired effect of the drug and extend its half-life, e.g. treatment with the organic acid probenecid can cause an increase in serum penicillin concentrations and hence allow a reduced frequency of administration.

See Case 14.1:2.

Drug dosing in renal failure

It is clear that Mrs Johnson had pre-existing renal impairment. Although her baseline serum creatinine was only

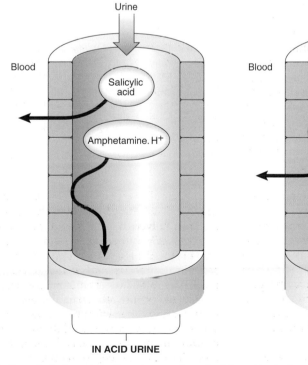

Fig. 14.4 Schematic of effect of altering urine pH on the excretion of acidic and basic drugs.

Drugs and the kidney: 2

Follow-up on Mrs Johnson

The results of Mrs Johnson's blood tests come back, indicating that the serum digoxin level (taken some 8h after the last dose) is 3.9 nmol/L. This is well outside the recommended therapeutic range (0.6–2.3 nmol/L) and, taken in conjunction with her clinical features, is indicative of digoxin toxicity.

Furthermore, her plasma biochemistry results now show some further deterioration in renal function, with the urea being *12.1 mmol/L and the creatinine *0.16 mmol/L. These results suggest that her poor fluid intake (due to nausea), in addition to her vomiting, have led to plasma volume contraction with a fall in renal blood flow and hence in GFR. This worsening renal impairment in turn would have led to further digoxin accumulation, setting up a vicious cycle of deterioration in her condition. Apart from the unpleasant gastrointestinal features experienced by this patient, other toxic effects of digoxin include visual disturbances and cardiac arrhythmias. The latter may be quite serious and are exacerbated by low plasma potassium levels which may occur as a result of diuretic therapy and/or vomiting in this setting.

Fortunately, with temporary cessation of digoxin and restoration of her hydration state, Mrs Johnson's digoxin toxicity state subsided, and she was later stabilized on a smaller daily dose of the drug (0.0625 mg).

It is now worth reviewing some of the factors which led Mrs Johnson into so much trouble.

* Values outside the normal range; see Appendix.

just outside the normal range, it can be shown by using the Cockroft–Gault formula (see Chapter 5) that her GFR was considerably reduced, at around 29 mL/min, when she first presented to hospital. Thus the dose and/or dosage interval of drugs such as digoxin (that are very largely excreted by the kidney) should have been modified to avoid accumulation and the attendant risk of toxicity. This risk should be considered before the administration of any drug to a patient with renal impairment, and any adverse reaction occurring in temporal relationship to a drug being started should be considered as being caused by the drug unless another explanation can be found.

Several characteristics of a drug suggest that there is a need for dosage adjustment and an increased risk of toxicity when the drug is prescribed for patients with renal impairment (Table 14.2). Some of these points have already arisen in the discussion about the case of Mrs Johnson.

Numerous published tables and algorithms are available to guide the therapeutic use of a wide variety of drugs in patients with different degrees of renal failure. Some examples are given in this chapter but further details can be obtained from reference texts.

Table 14.2 Characteristics of drugs that predict that a dosage adjustment should be made in renal disease

1. Primary urinary excretion of the parent drug or metabolites
In general, if greater than 50% of a drug or its active metabolites is normally excreted in the urine, a dosage reduction will be necessary to prevent accumulation and potential toxicity (e.g. gentamicin, allopurinol).

2. Low therapeutic index
Because of a narrow therapeutic range of efficacy of the drug, accumulation will result in significant toxicity (e.g. digoxin).

3. High protein binding
Accumulation of organic acids in chronic kidney disease will displace acidic drugs from albumin and increase free drug in the plasma, so that the target therapeutic concentration range (measuring total drug) should be adjusted downwards (e.g. phenytoin).

4. A small volume of distribution of the drug
Changes in body water that occur in renal disease are more likely to impact on drugs that are distributed in smaller volumes (e.g. highly protein-bound drugs).

Part B

Renal impairment induced by drugs

Drugs and the kidney: 1

A predictable reaction

Roger Woodruffe is a 60-year-old man who presents with recent pain in his left knee joint that has limited his golfing activities. He has a history of hypertension, well controlled on a combination of an angiotensin-converting enzyme (ACE) inhibitor (perindopril 4 mg/day) and a loop diuretic (furosemide [frusemide] 40 mg/day). He is otherwise well. His blood pressure at the time he is seen is 145/95 mm Hg. His serum biochemistry was last measured 6 months ago with the following results:

Sodium 140 mmol/L
Potassium 5.0 mmol/L
Chloride 105 mmol/L
Bicarbonate 23 mmol/L
*Urea 12.1 mmol/L
*Creatinine 0.16 mmol/L.

His doctor prescribes a non-steroidal anti-inflammatory drug (NSAID), diclofenac, 50 mg twice daily.

Mr Woodruffe returns for review in 10 days complaining of ankle swelling and mild dyspnoea on exertion. His blood pressure is now 175/105 mm Hg and he has pitting oedema bilaterally. His doctor orders a new serum biochemical profile which shows the creatinine has risen to *0.24 mmol/L and the potassium is now elevated at *6.6mmol/L. The serum albumin is normal at 41g/L. Urinalysis shows only a trace of protein, and a midstream urine specimen reveals no increased excretion of cells and no bacterial growth. A full blood count is normal, with no increased eosinophil count to suggest that an allergic reaction is involved.

This case raises the issues associated with prescribing drugs with predictable effects on renal haemodynamics and transport for patients with already impaired renal function. By understanding the relevant physiology and pharmacology, it will become clear that Mr Woodruffe was at high risk of renal functional deterioration from the prescription of the NSAID diclofenac.

* Values outside the normal range; see Appendix.

Renal actions of non-steroidal anti-inflammatory drugs

NSAIDs inhibit the formation of prostaglandins through the inhibition of cyclo-oxygenase (COX). Prostaglandins have a vasodilatory effect in the kidney, which is of particular significance in the presence of renal impairment. In this situation, glomerular filtration is maintained by increasing renal blood flow through afferent arteriolar vasodilatation (mediated by prostaglandins) and efferent arteriolar vasoconstriction (mediated by angiotensin II). Blockade of these compensatory mechanisms to maintain renal blood flow and GFR will be reflected by an increase in serum creatinine. Thus, prescription of NSAIDs in the presence of pre-existing renal impairment will commonly aggravate the degree of renal failure. This effect is exacerbated by concomitant use of ACE inhibitors and diuretics, which will further reduce the glomerular pressure and thus the driving force for glomerular filtration (see Chapter 5).

As prostaglandins also promote natriuresis by interfering with tubular sodium reabsorption, and blunt the effects of antidiuretic hormone on the tubular reabsorption of water, inhibition of prostaglandin production by NSAIDs results in salt and water retention, with resultant hypertension and oedema. Inhibition of prostaglandin synthesis also secondarily inhibits renin release, causing hyporeninaemic hypoaldosteronism which results in the impairment of distal tubular potassium secretion and hence hyperkalaemia. As these effects are caused by alterations in 'normal' physiological function, the urinalysis is unremarkable (minimal proteinuria or haematuria) and the urinary sediment is bland. In general, the abnormalities are corrected by withdrawal of the NSAID and any additional drugs affecting plasma volume and glomerular haemodynamics.

In summary, it is likely that all of Mr Woodruffe's problems at his second presentation – the worsening of renal function and hypertension, fluid retention and hyperkalaemia – are caused by the inhibition of renal COX by the NSAID diclofenac.

COX exists in two isoforms. COX 1 is constitutively expressed in the kidney and gastrointestinal tract, while COX 2 is expressed in inflamed tissues. Recently, drugs which selectively inhibit COX 2 have been developed for use in inflammatory conditions with the expectation that the side effect profile will be better than for the previously available non-selective COX 1 and 2 inhibitors. However, experience to date suggests that, while gastrointestinal side effects with the selective COX 2 inhibitors are greatly reduced, the effects on renal function and electrolyte homeostasis are comparable to the non-selective agents.

Case 14.2 Drugs and the kidney: 2

Course and outcome

Mr Woodruffe is advised to cease the diclofenac, furosemide (frusemide) and perindopril, and is changed to sustained-release verapamil 240mg/day as a replacement antihypertensive.

After 1 week, his oedema has largely resolved, the blood pressure has improved to 150/90 and his serum creatinine has fallen to *0.17mmol/L, with normal electrolytes.

* Values outside the normal range; see Appendix.

Mechanisms of nephrotoxicity

It is clear from the above case that drug-induced nephrotoxicity may be mediated by alterations in renal haemodynamics via an effect on humoral systems within the kidney. However, drugs may also be directly nephrotoxic to renal cells (largely affecting the tubular cells) or cause immunologically mediated damage. Thus a drug may directly induce acute tubular necrosis (although haemodynamic influences may also be involved), or trigger interstitial nephritis or, occasionally, glomerular injury.

Both of these latter mechanisms may be invoked in different patients in the nephrotoxicity observed with NSAIDs, in addition to the physiologically predictable haemodynamic and tubular transport effects noted above. In particular, NSAID-induced interstitial nephritis is seen relatively commonly, partly because of the high prevalence of usage in the community.

Drug-induced interstitial nephritis

Idiosyncratic responses to many drugs may include an acute interstitial nephritis. Because of the inflammatory nature of the condition, characterized by an interstitial inflammatory response with eosinophilic infiltration (Fig. 14.5), the urinalysis will generally show haematuria and proteinuria and often granular casts on urine microscopy. Renal function will generally deteriorate because of interstitial inflammation and oedema, causing a reduction in renal blood flow and GFR. The inflammatory cell infiltrate consists of a variety of cells, including B and T lymphocytes, plasma cells, natural killer cells and macrophages. In the majority of instances where T cell subsets have been studied in drug-induced interstitial nephritis, the CD4 population predominates. Peripheral eosinophilia is often present and, in occasional cases, a more systemic 'allergic' response will result in skin rashes and arthralgia. NSAIDs have been well documented to cause interstitial nephritis up to 6 months after stable therapy. However, in Mr Woodruffe's case, the diagnosis of interstitial nephritis is not supported, as the urinalysis and urine sediment were not abnormal and systemic features were not prominent.

Many drugs have been implicated as a cause of acute interstitial nephritis (Table 14.3), which can arise within a variable period from commencement of the drug. Thus, a deterioration in renal function in this setting should alert the clinician to the possibility of this diagnosis.

Fig. 14.5 Micrograph (stained with haematoxylin and eosin) showing acute interstitial nephritis. Note the intense inflammatory infiltrate and oedema in the interstitium; numerous eosinophils can be detected under high power.

Table 14.3 Drugs frequently implicated in acute interstitial nephritis

Antibiotics	**Others**
Penicillins (especially meticillin)	Phenytoin
Cephalosporins	Allopurinol
Sulphonamides	Aspirin
Rifampicin	Methyldopa
Quinolones	Carbamazepine
	Valproic acid
Diuretics	Diazepam
Thiazides	Interferon
Furosemide (frusemide)	Beta-blockers
	Quinine
NSAIDs	Doxepin
	Azathioprine

An improvement in renal function will generally follow the withdrawal of the offending agent. The time to recovery may vary from days to months. Renal biopsy is usually performed to confirm the diagnosis where there is

severe renal impairment, or because of systemic features which raise the question of **vasculitis**. In these cases, short-term treatment with corticosteroids may be of benefit in shortening the natural course of the illness. Although in the majority of cases GFR returns to baseline values, there is a loss of functional renal tissue in many cases, characterized histologically by interstitial fibrosis and sometimes glomerulosclerosis. Factors associated with a greater loss of renal functional capacity include more severe initial renal failure, a slower rate of recovery after withdrawal of the offending agent, greater histological damage, older age group and lack of initial steroid therapy.

Drug-induced glomerular pathology

Glomerular pathology is less common than tubulointerstitial injury in drug-induced nephrotoxicity. In general, glomerular damage presents as proteinuria and the most frequently observed pathology is membranous nephropathy. The frequency with which glomerular injury occurs in patients treated with certain drugs, notably gold and penicillamine (used mainly in rheumatoid arthritis), is high enough to warrant routine surveillance by urinalysis. In general, the prognosis of the glomerular lesion is favourable after withdrawal of the drug, with an improvement in proteinuria generally observed. The occurrence of **glomerulopathy** in this setting is not clearly dose-related, and the aetiology remains unclear.

NSAIDs may also induce a glomerulopathy, with minimal change nephropathy being the most widely recognized pathological lesion. However, this is rare, and is unlikely to be implicated in the deteriorating renal function in the case reviewed in the current chapter, as proteinuria was not present on urinalysis.

Important causes of nephrotoxicity

In the case of some drugs, nephrotoxicity may be dose-related and predictable, while in other cases the condition is an uncommon side effect, but may be frequently observed if there is a high usage of the particular agent in the community. Some examples of common or important causes of nephrotoxicity are discussed below.

Gentamicin

Gentamicin (and other aminoglycosides) require specific mention because of the serious and avoidable nature of the toxicity associated with this class of antibiotics. Aminoglycosides are almost entirely excreted by the kidney. Thus, in renal failure excretion of the drug is reduced and, unless dosage modification is made, toxicity is likely to occur, affecting both the kidney and inner ear. The effectiveness of an aminoglycoside in killing bacteria correlates with its peak concentration rather than with its steady state concentration, whereas the nephrotoxicity correlates with the steady state accumulation of the drug into proximal tubular cells. Thus, in renal failure the drug dosage remains the same but the dose interval should be increased. In patients with end-stage renal failure, where the only clearance is through the dialysis process, the dose interval may be up to every 3 days. This contrasts with agents such as digoxin (and cyclosporin, discussed below) where a therapeutic effect requires a defined steady state concentration to be maintained. In these cases the dose is reduced but the dosage interval remains constant.

In patients with any degree of renal impairment, the clearance of a renally excreted drug may be hard to predict. Thus, whenever accumulation of a drug poses a predictable risk of toxicity, serum concentrations of the drug just before the next scheduled dose (trough level) should be used to guide either the dose or the dosage interval, as appropriate.

Cyclosporin

Cyclosporin A is an immunosuppressive drug which is largely metabolized in the liver, but the main clinical manifestation of toxicity is renal injury. Several mechanisms of toxicity are recognized. Cyclosporin A induces marked intrarenal vasoconstriction and a fall in GFR, with acute damage to the proximal tubules and ischaemic nephropathy in the longer term. A classic histological appearance of 'striped fibrosis' occurs in chronic cyclosporin nephrotoxicity. An **arteriopathy** is also well recognized with a syndrome consistent with haemolytic uraemic syndrome, characterized by activation of the coagulation system and intravascular haemolysis, resulting in anaemia, **thrombocytopenia** and impaired renal function.

As cyclosporin A is metabolized by the cytochrome-dependent mixed function oxidases in the liver, drugs which interact with this system may impair its metabolism, thus precipitating significant toxicity or, alternatively, accelerate metabolism resulting in loss of the immunosuppressive effect. As cyclosporin is widely used in renal transplantation, drug levels are closely monitored as fluctuations in renal function in this circumstance are common and a high cyclosporin level may provide evidence suggesting the development of nephrotoxicity.

Renal disease induced by non-prescription medicines

Epidemiological studies have clearly identified the ingestion of aspirin, phenacetin and caffeine in over-the-counter compound analgesic medications as a cause of a characteristic interstitial nephritis with **papillary necrosis**, associated with an increased propensity to uroepithelial carcinoma. This clinical entity of *analgesic nephropathy* has been the most prevalent clearly recognized cause of drug-induced end-stage renal failure within defined demographic populations (including Australia). Although analgesic nephropathy accounted for up to 22% of patients entering dialysis programs in the early 1980s, its incidence has steadily declined since the withdrawal of these medications in combination form from over-the-counter sale. Long-term ingestion of NSAIDs has been implicated in the pathogenesis of some cases of interstitial nephritis and papillary necrosis. However, the incidence is relatively low compared with the former usage of the compound agents.

'Natural' therapies are increasingly being used for a variety of conditions in both western and eastern cultures. The constituents of such therapies are often poorly documented, and they may result in either dose-dependent or idiosyncratic side effects. One recently reported form of so-called 'Chinese Herb Nephropathy' related to the use of *Aristolochia frangchi* for weight reduction. This has been causally demonstrated to induce a rapidly progressive non-inflammatory interstitial fibrosis in the kidney, resulting in end-stage kidney disease. Follow-up investigations in these patients have revealed an increased risk of uroepithelial cancer, high enough to justify recommendation of prophylactic nephrectomy before consideration of transplantation and immunosuppression.

Contrast agents

Intravenous administration of iodinated radiological contrast agents has been reported to be nephrotoxic, particularly in patients with volume depletion, pre-existing renal disease, diabetes mellitus or multiple myeloma. In general, an acute reversible decline in renal function is observed and, in severe cases, the underlying pathological lesion is acute tubular necrosis. The newer non-ionic compounds have been reported to be less nephrotoxic and are preferred, particularly in high-risk patients. It is recommended that intravenous saline loading be undertaken in these patients before the procedure, since this measure has been found to be protective in laboratory and clinical studies. Furthermore, agents that may exacerbate renal haemodynamic injury, such as NSAIDs and ACE inhibitors, should be ceased. In many instances, alternative means of imaging can now be undertaken, and these should be carefully considered in patients with advanced renal disease.

The ranges shown are for adults unless otherwise stated.

	Range	Units
Haematology		
Haemoglobin (men)	130–180	g/L
(women)	115–165	g/L
White cell count	4.0–11.0	$\times 10^9$/L
Platelet count	150–400	$\times 10^9$/L
Packed cell volume (haematocrit)	0.38–0.52	
Erythrocyte sedimentation rate	3–15	mm/h
Biochemistry		
Venous plasma or serum		
Sodium (Na)	135–145	mmol/L
Potassium (K)	3.5–5.0	mmol/L
Chloride (Cl)	95–110	mmol/L
Bicarbonate (HCO_3^- or 'total CO_2')	22–30	mmol/L
Urea	3.0–8.0	mmol/L
Creatinine (adults)	0.06–0.12	mmol/L
(children)	0.03–0.08	mmol/L
Osmolality	280–300	mosm/kg water
Glucose ('BSL') (fasting)	3.0–5.4	mmol/L
(random)	3.0–7.7	mmol/L
HbA_{1C}	3.5–6.0	%
Total protein	62–80	g/L
Albumin	32–45	g/L
Total calcium (Ca)	2.10–2.60	mmol/L
Phosphate (PO_4)	0.8–1.5	mmol/L
Magnesium (Mg)	0.8–1.0	mmol/L
Urate	0.2–0.4	mmol/L
Total cholesterol	<5.5	mmol/L
Triglycerides (fasting)	<2.0	mmol/L
Arterial blood		
pO_2	80–105	mm Hg
pCO_2	35–45	mm Hg
pH	7.36–7.44	
HCO_3^-	22–30	mmol/L
Urine		
Protein	<150	mg/24 h
Urate	2.0–6.6	mmol/24 h
Calcium	2.5–7.5	mmol/24 h
Creatinine (depends on muscle mass)	6–16	mmol/24 h
Sodium (depends on intake)	50–200	mmol/24 h
Potassium (depends on intake)	40–100	mmol/24 h
Osmolality (depends on hydration)	50–1200	mosm/kg water
Immunology		
Antinuclear antibodies (ANA)	1:100 or less	
dsDNA antibodies	<7	IU/mL
Complement:		
C3	0.75–1.75	g/L
C4	0.10 0.40	g/L
Microbiology		
Midstream urine – microscopy and culture		
White blood cells	<10	$\times 10^6$/L
Red blood cells	<10	$\times 10^6$/L
Epithelial cells	<10	$\times 10^6$/L
Bacterial colony count	$<10^7$	/L

systemic lupus erythematosus (SLE) – an autoimmune inflammatory disorder affecting multiple body systems.

thrombocytopenia – an abnormally low platelet count in the blood.

tubulo-interstitium – the component of the kidney parenchyma consisting of the tubules and the interstitial tissue.

tumour lysis syndrome – condition resulting from the rapid breakdown of malignant tissue, typically after chemotherapy.

uraemia (uraemic syndrome) – a biochemical and clinical state associated with the presence of large amounts of urea and other nitrogenous waste products in the blood, as occurs in advanced renal failure.

urinalysis – a chemical examination of the urine, most commonly performed using a dipstick containing reagents impregnated on paper squares.

Index